GW00374163

DEPARTMENT OF TRANSPORT

Transport Statistics Report

ROAD ACCIDENT STATISTICS ENGLISH REGIONS 1993

Published August 1994

London: HMSO

Brief extracts from this publication may be reproduced provided the source is fully acknowledged. Proposals for reproduction of larger extracts should be addressed to the Copyright Section, Her Majesty's Stationery Office, St Crispins, Duke Street, Norwich NR3 1PD.

Prepared for publication by STD5 branch
Directorate of Statistics
Department of Transport

Richard Ackroyd
Paul O'Connor
Linden Francis

GOVERNMENT STATISTICAL SERVICE

A service of statistical information and advice is provided to the government by specialist staff employed in the statistics divisions of individual Departments. Statistics are made generally available through their publications and further information and advice on them can be obtained from the Departments concerned.

Enquiries about the contents of this publication should be made to:

**Directorate of Statistics
Department of Transport
Room B648
Romney House
43 Marsham Street
London SW1P 3PY**

Telephone 071 276 8785

Data Service

Copies of the main tables in this publication can be supplied on a computer diskette by the Department of Transport (at a cost of £40). Further tabulations of road accident statistics are also available from the Department, subject to confidentiality rules. The charges vary with the complexity of the analysis (minimum £40) and the availability of these services depends upon the resources within the Department. Enquiries should be addressed in writing to Mr P S O'Connor at the above address

Contents

Symbols and Conventions

Rounding of Figures:

In tables where figures have been rounded there may be an apparent slight discrepancy between the sum of the constituent items and the independently rounded total.

Symbols:

'..' = not available

Conversion Factor:

1 kilometre = 0.6214 mile

Preface

This is the 1993 edition of Road Accident Statistics English Regions (RASER), a publication which gives statistics of road accidents on a local basis for England. RASER concentrates on accidents as being incidents which may reflect a need for local action and is intended to be of most benefit to traffic engineers, planners and administrators in local government and the Department of Transport (DOT) regional offices. For this reason, most of the data in the book are compiled according to the county groupings covered by these offices (which are shown on the map on the next page).

RASER is confined to background national statistics, so it should be regarded as a supplement to 'Road Accidents Great Britain 1993 - The Casualty Report' (RAGB), which is the main publication on road accident statistics in Great Britain. RAGB 1993 is available from HMSO bookshops, price £11.25.

The current system of collecting road accident statistics was set up in 1968, and is for the benefit and use of local authorities, the police and central government. Each year, about 230,000 STATS19 road accident report forms (an example of which can be found on pages 45 to 47) are completed by police officers of the 51 police forces in Great Britain. These forms record data about accidents on the public highway which involved personal injury or death. These data are transferred onto magnetic tape or computer diskette and are sent to DOT where they are incorporated into an annual data file.

The principal purpose in collecting and publishing statistics of road accidents is to provide background information for both central government and local authorities on the roads, road users, places, times of day, weather conditions, where road accidents happen etc, and against which various remedial measures can be considered. Road accident statistics are used to provide both a local and a national perspective for particular road safety problems or particular suggested remedies. A continuous flow of information - such as the time series tables in this book - means that trends of accidents and casualties can be examined and used to change the direction of policies when necessary.

The report also includes data from Northern Ireland. These data, where available, are included with each table along with data for Scotland and Wales. *More detailed statistics for Scotland and Wales are available from the Scottish and Welsh Offices - please refer to the inside rear cover for more details.*

Several of the tables contain averages of 1981-85 data. These represent the base figures which the Secretary of State for Transport used to set the target of reducing the number of road casualties by one third by the year 2000. It should also be noted that main Tables 1 and 6 which give casualty totals by severity for the years covering 1981 to 1985 have been extended to show revised estimates for London for this period. At the beginning of September 1984 the Metropolitan police implemented improved procedures for allocating the level of severity to accidents and casualties. The change is thought to have had no effect on overall casualty numbers, but in the period between 1981 and the date of the change it is estimated that there were 4,725 casualties whose injuries were originally judged to be slight but would have been judged serious under the later procedures. However, this is an overall estimate and it is not possible to present similar revised estimates of accidents by road type and other detailed characteristics.

DOT is generally prepared to sell tabulations of road accident data. The cost of data varies with the complexity of each request, but averages about £40 per year of data. Further information can be obtained from: - *Mr Paul O'Connor, Department of Transport, Room B648, Romney House, 43 Marsham Street, London SW1P 3PY, Telephone 071-276-8785.*

DEPARTMENT OF TRANSPORT REGIONAL ORGANISATION

AS AT NOVEMBER 1991

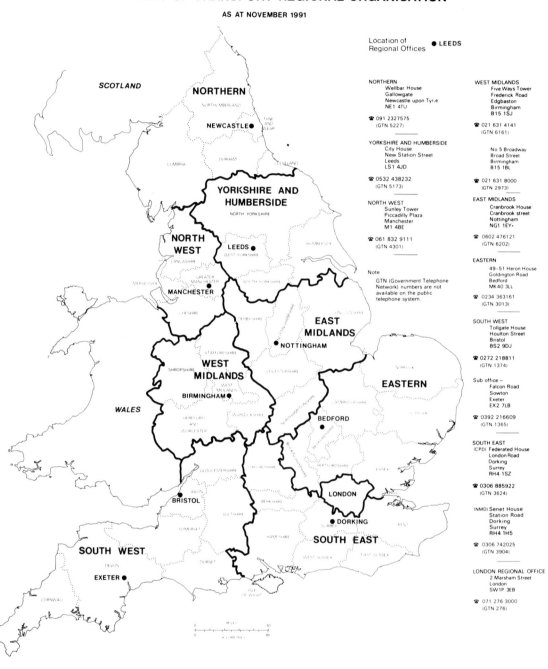

Location of Regional Offices ● LEEDS

NORTHERN
Wellbar House
Gallowgate
Newcastle upon Tyne
NE1 4TU
☎ 091 2327575
(GTN 5227)

YORKSHIRE AND HUMBERSIDE
City House
New Station Street
Leeds
LS1 4JD
☎ 0532 438232
(GTN 5173)

NORTH WEST
Sunley Tower
Piccadilly Plaza
Manchester
M1 4BE
☎ 061 832 9111
(GTN 4301)

Note
GTN (Government Telephone Network) numbers are not available on the public telephone system.

WEST MIDLANDS
Five Ways Tower
Frederick Road
Edgbaston
Birmingham
B15 1SJ
☎ 021 631 4141
(GTN 6161)

No 5 Broadway
Broad Street
Birmingham
B15 1BL
☎ 021 631 8000
(GTN 2973)

EAST MIDLANDS
Cranbrook House
Cranbrook street
Nottingham
NG1 1EY·
☎ 0602 476121
(GTN 6202)

EASTERN
49–51 Heron House
Goldington Road
Bedford
MK40 3LL
☎ 0234 363161
(GTN 3013)

SOUTH WEST
Tollgate House
Houlton Street
Bristol
BS2 9DJ
☎ 0272 218811
(GTN 1374)

Sub office:—
Falcon Road
Sowton
Exeter
EX2 7LB
☎ 0392 216609
(GTN 1365)

SOUTH EAST
(CPD) Federated House
London Road
Dorking
Surrey
RH4 1SZ
☎ 0306 885922
(GTN 3624)

(NMD) Senet House
Station Road
Dorking
Surrey
RH4 1H5
☎ 0306 742025
(GTN 3904)

LONDON REGIONAL OFFICE
2 Marsham Street
London
SW1P 3EB
☎ 071 276 3000
(GTN 276)

Further copies of this map may be obtained from:
HGU Drawing Office
P2/019, 2 Marsham St.

Department of Transport
HGU Drawing Office 91 198

1. Commentary on tables and charts

Richard Ackroyd

1.1 Introduction

This section gives a review of the main body of tables included in this report. As noted in the introduction, the data in most of the tables are disaggregated either by county or Department of Transport (DOT) region and Northern Ireland data have been included within certain tables. Tables where Northern Ireland data are not available, and thus where no United Kingdom total can be given, have been individually annotated.

As reported last year in *Road Accident Statistics English Regions 1992*, from 1 April 1991 responsibility for the county of Cumbria transferred from the North West region of the DOT organisation to the Northern region. The DOT accident database was amended with effect from 1 January 1992 and as a consequence the numbers and rates for 1992 and 1993 as shown in this report have been based on the new organisation, but for the years up to and including 1991 the old definition has been used.

In order to provide consistent time series, the casualty data for the Northern and North West regions in Table 1 (page 21) have been calculated throughout according to the new definitions and these times series are also shown in the table below. The data for previous years in these two regions in Table 14 have also been similarly revised. However, the change in definitions means that in the remaining tables the 1992 and 1993 data for these regions are not consistent with data for previous years.

Casualties: Northern and North West regions by severity: 1981-1985 average, 1987-1993

								number
	1981−5 average	1987	1988	1989	1990	1991	1992	1993
Northern[1]								
Killed	282	294	280	270	334	287	225	230
Killed or seriously injured	3,466	2,916	2,947	2,962	3,050	2,651	2,475	2,178
All casualties	13,913	13,858	14,029	15,597	16,021	14,848	14,468	13,880
North West[2]								
Killed	538	522	498	512	487	468	437	379
Killed or seriously injured	6,219	5,391	5,172	5,334	5,470	4,972	4,811	4,705
All casualties	33,478	35,183	36,375	39,203	40,729	39,014	40,445	40,510

1. Including Cumbria − see above text.
2. Excluding Cumbria − see above text.

1.2 Casualties

Table 1 gives the regional distribution of casualties and is presented as a time series for the period 1987 to 1993. The average for the years 1981-1985 is also given. There has been little significant change in the aggregate casualty distribution between the regions over this period.

In each of the seven years shown, London had the highest number of casualties. In the years 1987 to 1990 the next highest number of casualties was in the South East region but since 1991 the next highest number was in the North West region. The lowest number of casualties was in the Northern region, which had, under the old regional definition, and until 1991, about half those in the East Midland region, the next lowest in England. Under the revised regional definition, this proportion has fallen to a little over one third.

The table also shows that in 1993, as in previous years, London had the highest overall casualty rate per 100,000 population, followed by the North West and Eastern regions. The lowest rates were found in the Northern and South West regions. London, however, had the lowest fatality rate of all the regions - probably because accidents in urban areas tend to be less severe because they occur at lower speeds. The highest fatality rate was in the East Midlands region with the next highest in the Eastern and Yorkshire & Humberside regions.

Chart 1a depicts the number of casualties killed and the number seriously injured in each region in 1993. The chart shows that the South East and Eastern regions had the highest number of those killed and London the highest number of those seriously injured.

Chart 1b depicts the number of casualties killed or seriously injured (KSI) and slightly injured in each region in 1993 and shows that London had the highest number of casualties in both severity groups and the Northern region and Wales the lowest number.

Chart 2 depicts the number of child (aged 0-15) casualties per 100,000 child population in each region in 1993 and shows that Scotland had the highest rate of children killed or seriously injured and the South East and South West regions the lowest rate. The North West region had the highest overall rate of child casualties. **Chart 3** shows the number of adult casualties per 100,000 population in each region in 1993 and shows that the Eastern and East Midlands regions had the highest rate of adults killed or seriously injured and the Northern region the lowest rate. The North West and London regions had the highest overall rate of adult casualties.

Charts 4 and **5** depict the percentage change in overall casualties and those killed or seriously injured for each region between 1992 and 1993 (the charts take account of the change in regional definition as noted in the introduction). **Chart 4** shows that overall casualties have fallen in six of the English regions and in Scotland and Wales. Scotland had the largest fall, at 7 per cent, and in England the Northern region had the largest fall, at 4 per cent. Casualties remained virtually unchanged in two English regions, and rose in one, the South West, by 2 per cent. **Chart 5** shows that casualties killed or seriously injured fell in every English region and in Scotland and Wales. The largest fall was in Scotland and Wales, both at 14 per cent, and amongst English regions the largest fall was in the Northern region, at 12 per cent.

1.3 Local authority casualty comparisons

Tables 2-5 give information on the number of casualties, rate per 100,000 population, and percentage distribution, by age and road user type for each English county, Scotland and Wales.

Table 2 gives the number of casualties by age and road user type for 1993 and **Table 3** gives the same information as an average for the years 1981-1985.

Table 4 gives casualty rates, per 100,000 population, by age and by type of road user for each English county. In England in 1993, 373 children were killed or injured in road accidents per 100,000 children and the county casualty rates varied from 248 in Avon to 552 in Merseyside. The casualty rate for those aged 60 and over varied from 185 in Avon to 362 in Greater London. The overall casualty rate for all ages was lowest in Avon and highest in Merseyside. The pedestrian casualty rate was highest in most urbanised areas, in particular London, Greater Manchester and Merseyside, and lowest in rural counties such as Shropshire and West Sussex. The pedal cyclist casualty rate was highest in Cambridgeshire and lowest in Durham and Tyne & Wear. The car occupant casualty rate varied from 206 in Avon and Tyne & Wear to 481 in Merseyside.

Table 5 gives the distribution of casualties, by age and by type of road user, for each county. In England in 1993, 14 per cent of road accident casualties were children and 11 per cent were aged 60 and over. The proportion of casualties who were children varied from 10 per cent in Surrey to 20 per cent in Cleveland and Tyne & Wear. Dorset and East Sussex had the highest proportion of casualties aged 60 or over; 16 per cent compared with 11 per cent in the whole of England.

Table 6 gives the number of casualties killed or seriously injured and total casualties in each English county for 1993 and compares them with the average for the years 1981-1985. The percentage change is also given. In England as a whole, the number killed or seriously has fallen by 38 per cent and overall casualties by 4 per cent. The number of casualties killed or seriously injured has fallen in every county, with the largest fall, at 65 per cent, in Berkshire.

1.4 Casualties by road type

Charts 6a and **6b** depict the number of casualties killed or seriously injured and slightly injured in each region on built-up and non built-up roads respectively. On built-up roads, the highest number of casualties for both severity groups was in London, with Wales and the Northern region having the lowest number for both severity groups. On non built-up roads, the highest number of casualties killed or seriously injured was in the Eastern region and the highest number of slight casualties was in the South East and Eastern regions. The lowest number of casualties for both severity groups was in London.

Table 7 gives the total number of casualties in each region disaggregated by severity and by road type. In each regions, over 50 per cent of casualties were in accidents on built-up roads and, except in the South East region with 6 per cent, no more than 5 per cent of casualties were in accidents on motorways. The proportion of casualties who were killed or seriously injured was highest on non-built up roads.

Charts 7 and **8** show, for built-up and non built-up roads respectively, overall casualty numbers on trunk, principal and 'other' roads in each region in 1993. On built-up roads, the highest number of casualties on trunk and principal roads was in London and the highest number of casualties on 'other' roads was in the North West region. On non built-up roads, the highest number of casualties on trunk roads and 'other' roads was in the Eastern region and the highest number of casualties on principal roads in the South East region.

Table 8 gives the casualty rates by severity for motorways and A roads for each region. The casualty rate is derived by dividing the number of casualties on a particular road type by the traffic carried on those roads. The rates are given as an average for the period 1991 to 1993.

The data show that the highest 'all severities' rate on motorways was in London, with the lowest in the South West region. London also had the highest 'all severities' rate for all A roads, and the South West the lowest rate. For England as a whole, the highest 'all severities' rate was on built-up trunk and principal roads, and the lowest on motorways.

1.5 Accidents

Table 9 gives accident rates by severity for motorways and A roads for each region. The accident rate is derived by dividing the number of accidents on particular road types by the traffic carried on that road type. The rates are given as an average for the period 1991 to 1993. The data show that over the three year period, in England as a whole, built-up principal A roads had the highest overall accident rate at 99 accidents per 100 million vehicle kilometres and motorways the lowest rate at 11 accidents per 100 million vehicle kilometres. For fatal accidents, the respective rates for these two road types were 1.2 accidents and 0.3 accidents. The table also shows that accident rates were higher on principal A roads than on trunk A roads.

Chart 9 depicts the number of accidents on motorways and trunk and principal A roads in each region in 1993. The chart shows that the South East region had the highest number of accidents on motorways, and London the highest number of accidents on trunk and principal A roads.

1.6 Seasonal pattern of accidents

The seasonal pattern of injury accidents is given in **Table 10**. The base has been calculated as the average number of accidents per day in each region. The peak months for accidents can vary from year to year for various reasons, for example, differing weather conditions. The general pattern is low accident numbers in the early part of the year, gradually building up to a peak in May, June and July, followed by a small dip and then a higher peak from October to December. This trend continued in 1993, when the peak month for all accidents was November or December in all English regions except the South West. February had the lowest number of accidents in all English regions except the Northern. When accident figures are related to the number of days in each month, the lowest daily rate of all accidents was in February or March in all English regions. The highest daily rate was in November or December in all English regions except again in the South West. The pattern for fatal and serious accidents differs slightly than that for all accidents, with the peak month for these accidents, both in number and by day, being December in four of the English regions and ranging from May to October in the remaining five regions.

1.7 Accidents by road type

Tables 11-13 show the number of junction and non-junction injury accidents occurring on motorways and trunk and principal A roads. On motorways in England, 16 per cent of accidents occurred at junctions and roundabouts. On trunk A roads, 58 per cent of accidents occurred at junctions and roundabouts as did 69 per cent of accidents on principal A roads.

Junction accidents, including those on roundabouts, accounted for about 50 per cent of all trunk A road accidents in each region except the West Midlands region where the proportion was higher at 61 per cent, and the North West and London regions, where the proportion rose to 67 and 69 per cent respectively. This pattern was repeated on principal A roads, where just over 60 per cent of accidents occurred at junctions in all regions except in the West Midlands and North West regions where the proportion rose to 69 and 74 per cent respectively and in London, where the proportion was 77 per cent.

Table 14 gives the total number of injury accidents disaggregated by severity on different types of road in each region and county for 1992 and 1993. The average for the years 1981 to 1985 is also given. The road classifications used are motorways, trunk and principal A roads and all roads.

Table 15 shows injury accidents and casualties by severity, and the vehicles involved, for individual English motorways, including A(M) roads. Eighty three per cent of the vehicles involved were cars or vans while 14 per cent were heavy lorries, broadly in line with their share of motorway traffic. Motorways with the highest numbers of accidents per kilometre in 1993 were the M25 (4.4 accidents), the M63 (3.3), and the M4 (3.2 accidents).

Table 16 gives the percentage of accidents on the various types of road within each region. This table should be considered in conjunction with Table 19 which shows the distribution of motor traffic within each region.

1.8 Background data

Table 17 gives regional background information on road lengths, home population, area, and licensed vehicle numbers. **Table 18** gives the 1991-1993 average distribution between regions of motor traffic on major roads, and **Table 19** shows the distribution of motor traffic within each region. The English motorway lengths shown in Tables 15 and 17 have been supplied by DOT Highways Computing Division from data extracted from the Network Information System (NIS). Other road lengths in Table 17 are taken from the Transport Statistics Report *'Road Lengths in Great Britain 1993'*.

List of charts and tables

CHARTS

Chart 1a: Fatal and serious casualties: by region: 1993

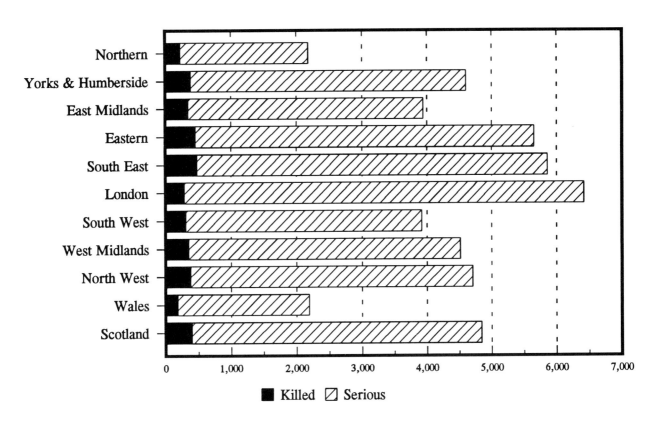

Chart 1b: KSI and slight casualties: by region: 1993

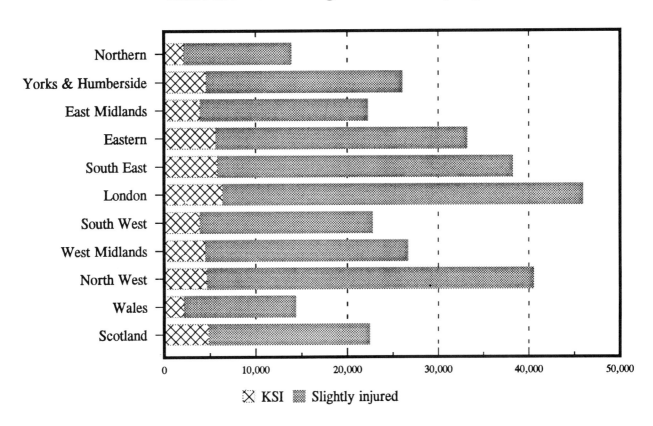

Chart 2: Child casualties per 100,000 population: by severity and region: 1993

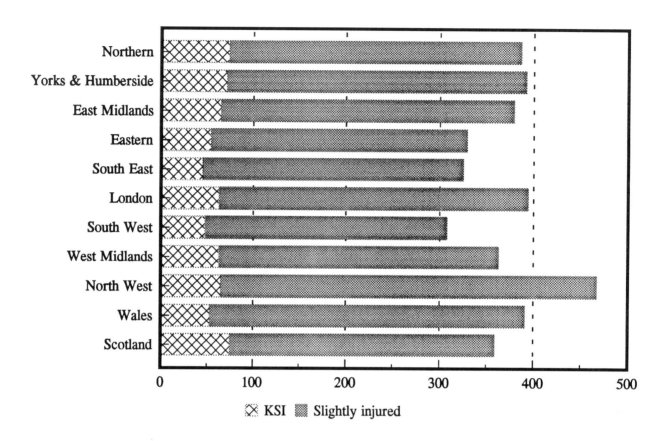

Chart 3: Adult casualties per 100,000 population: by severity and region: 1993

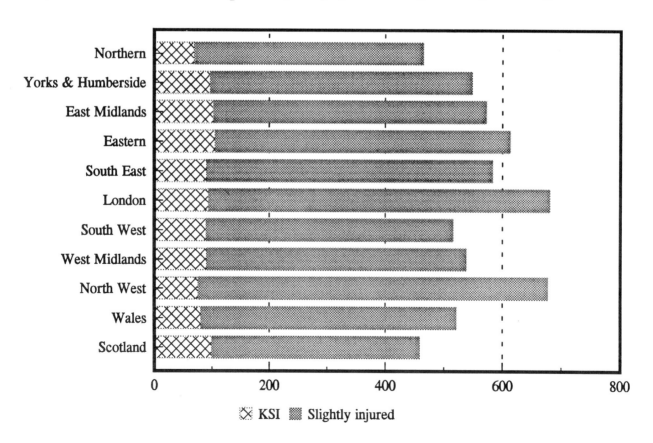

Chart 4: Percentage change in total casualties: by region: 1992-1993

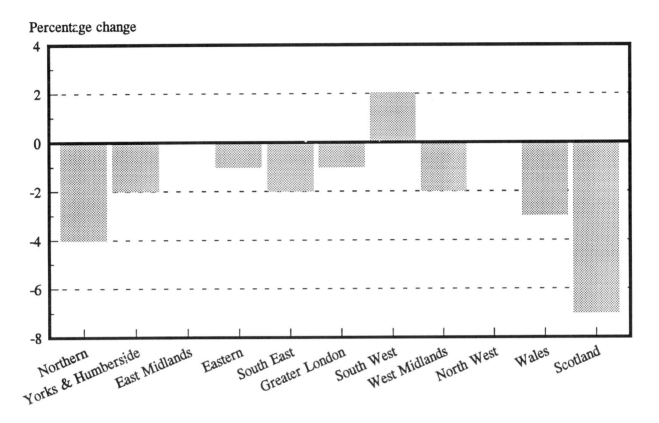

Chart 5: Percentage change in KSI casualties: by region: 1992-1993

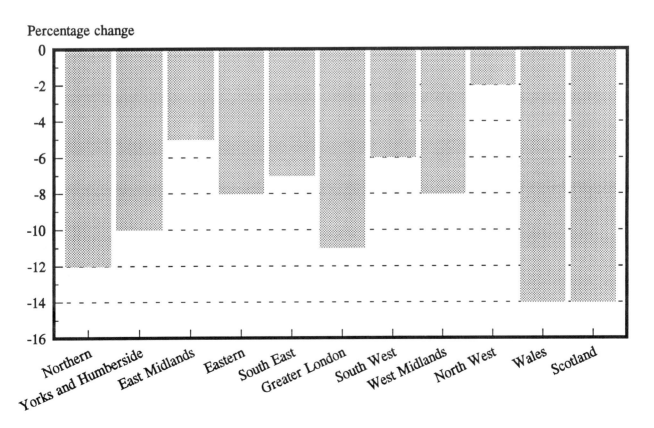

Chart 6a: Casualties on built-up roads: by severity and region: 1993

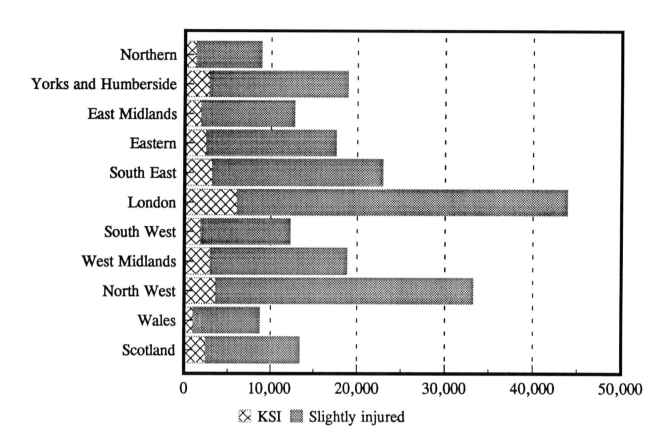

KSI ⊠ Slightly injured ▓

Chart 6b: Casualties on non built-up roads: by severity and region: 1993

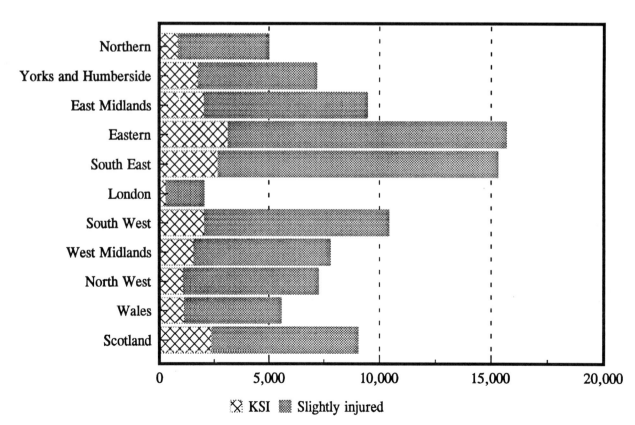

KSI ⊠ Slightly injured ▓

Chart 7: Casualties by road class and region: built-up roads: 1993

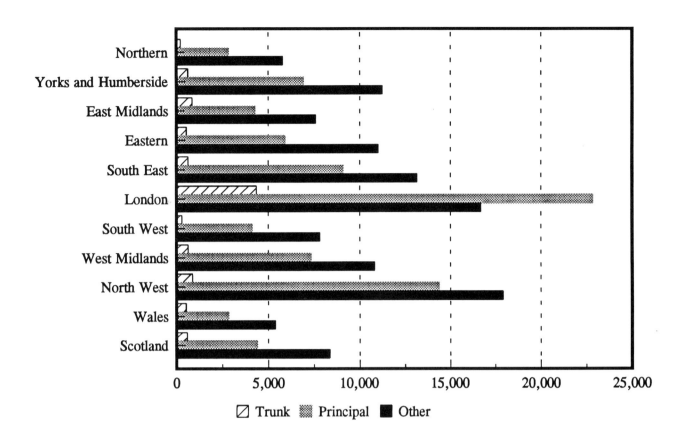

Trunk ▨   Principal ▨   Other ■

Chart 8: Casualties by road class and region: non built-up roads: 1993

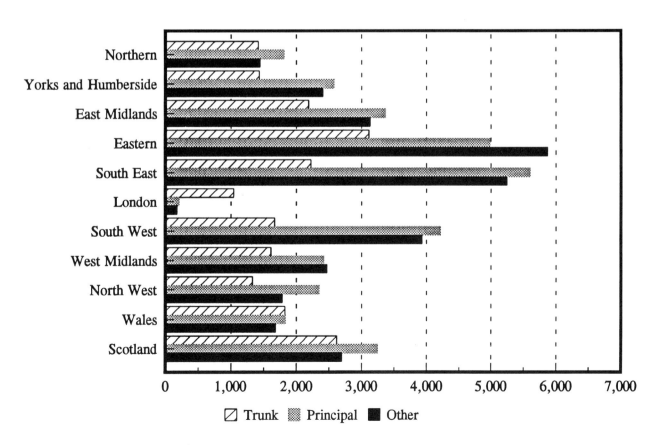

Trunk ▨   Principal ▨   Other ■

Chart 9: Accidents by road class and region: 1993

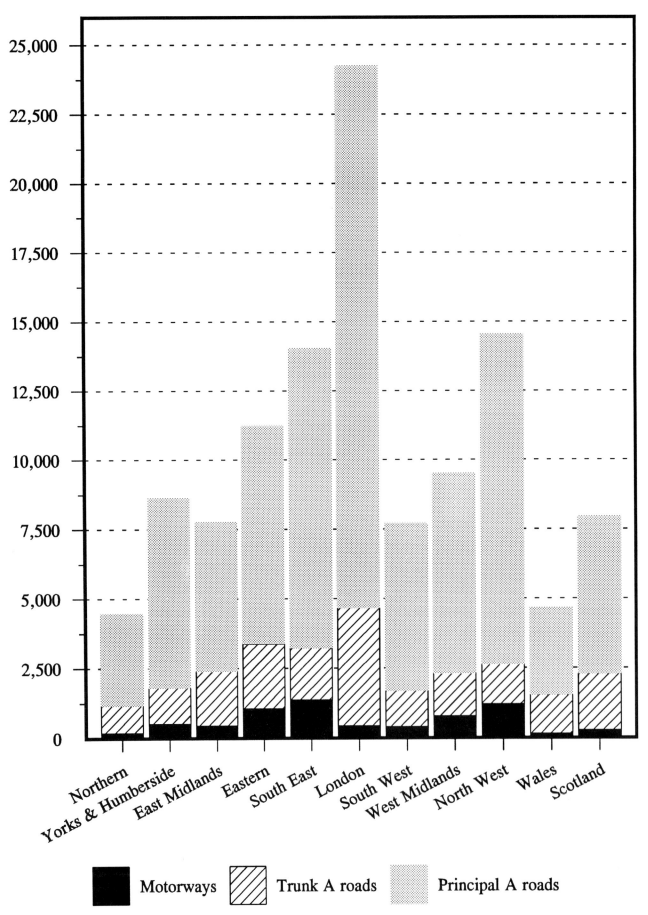

Motorways ▨ Trunk A roads ░ Principal A roads

TABLES

1 Casualties: by region and severity: 1981-85 average, 1987-1993: rate per 100,000 population, 1993

	1981-85 Average	1987	1988	1989	1990	1991	1992	1993	1993 Rate Per 100,000 Population[1]
Northern[2]									
Killed	282	294	280	270	334	287	225	230	7.4
Killed or seriously injured	3,566	2,916	2,947	2,962	3,050	2,651	2,475	2,178	70.3
All Casualties	13,913	13,858	14,029	15,597	16,021	14,848	14,468	13,880	447.9
Yorkshire and Humberside									
Killed	501	440	437	480	428	413	414	387	7.7
Killed or seriously injured	6,830	5,817	6,131	6,127	5,978	5,202	5,110	4,603	92.0
All Casualties	25,915	25,328	26,884	28,560	28,455	26,086	26,599	26,031	520.4
East Midlands									
Killed	492	448	413	514	513	410	393	350	8.6
Killed or seriously injured	6,389	5,254	5,031	5,342	5,045	4,173	4,145	3,940	97.0
All Casualties	23,079	22,494	23,308	25,129	24,852	22,397	22,175	22,207	546.7
Eastern									
Killed	601	614	587	617	608	546	488	455	7.8
Killed or seriously injured	9,312	8,318	8,230	7,967	7,653	6,287	6,132	5,656	97.2
All Casualties	33,789	35,886	37,896	39,424	37,908	33,768	33,388	33,180	570.0
South East									
Killed	735	676	718	715	699	516	496	478	6.8
Killed or seriously injured	11,038	9,446	9,321	8,766	8,155	6,388	6,325	5,859	82.9
All Casualties	41,999	40,326	41,184	43,050	42,387	38,211	38,876	38,225	540.9
London[3]									
Killed	539	456	446	460	408	368	316	286	4.1
Killed or seriously injured	8,230 (9,175)	9,517	9,478	9,344	8,910	7,878	7,233	6,419	93.0
All Casualties	54,156	49,454	50,114	52,779	51,871	46,578	46,417	45,927	665.2
South West									
Killed	484	457	462	521	468	460	385	310	6.5
Killed or seriously injured	8,047	6,250	6,134	5,781	5,424	4,555	4,153	3,916	82.5
All Casualties	26,352	24,507	25,444	25,246	25,034	22,515	22,302	22,728	478.9
West Midlands									
Killed	526	442	442	498	478	386	395	353	6.7
Killed or seriously injured	7,857	5,860	5,774	6,190	6,136	5,298	4,913	4,514	85.5
All Casualties	27,699	25,425	26,760	28,964	30,219	27,425	27,089	26,599	504.0
North West[2]									
Killed	538	522	498	512	487	468	437	379	5.9
Killed or seriously injured	6,219	5,391	5,172	5,334	5,470	4,972	4,811	4,705	73.5
All Casualties	33,478	35,183	36,375	39,203	40,729	39,014	40,445	40,510	633.0
England									
Killed	4,698	4,349	4,283	4,587	4,423	3,854	3,549	3,228	6.7
Killed or seriously injured	67,388	58,769	58,218	57,813	55,821	47,404	45,297	41,790	86.4
All Casualties	280,382	272,461	281,994	297,952	297,476	270,842	271,759	269,287	556.6
Wales									
Killed	259	220	226	233	249	227	220	187	6.5
Killed or seriously injured	3,855	3,388	3,127	3,191	3,037	2,638	2,537	2,189	75.5
All Casualties	14,395	14,266	15,164	16,165	16,432	15,074	14,732	14,331	494.4
Scotland									
Killed	641	556	543	553	545	487	460	399	7.8
Killed or seriously injured	8,887	7,261	7,198	7,527	6,800	6,131	5,640	4,844	94.8
All Casualties	27,134	24,746	25,147	27,475	27,233	25,353	24,182	22,402	438.3
Great Britain									
Killed	5,598	5,125	5,052	5,373	5,217	4,568	4,229	3,814	6.8
Killed or seriously injured	80,130	69,418	68,543	68,531	65,658	56,173	53,474	48,823	86.6
All Casualties	321,912	311,473	322,305	341,592	341,141	311,269	310,673	306,020	542.7
Northern Ireland									
Killed	196	214	178	181	185	185	150	143	8.9
Killed or seriously injured	2,362	2,099	2,147	2,195	2,178	1,833	1,991	1,725	107.1
All Casualties	8,204	9,936	10,967	11,611	11,761	10,314	11,264	11,100	689.3
United Kingdom									
Killed	5,793	5,339	5,230	5,554	5,402	4,753	4,379	3,957	6.8
Killed or seriously injured	82,492	71,517	70,690	70,726	67,836	58,006	55,465	50,548	87.2
All Casualties	330,115	321,409	333,272	353,203	352,902	321,583	321,937	317,120	546.8

1 Based on final 1992 population estimates.

2 From 1st April 1991 responsibilty for Cumbria transferred from the North West Regional Office to the Northern Regional Office. The change to the road accident database was deferred until 1992. Data prior to 1992 for both Northern and North West regions have been revised to take account of the change in boundaries (see introduction on page 3).

3. In September 1984 the Metropolitan Police implemented revised standards in the assessment of serious casualties. The figure in brackets is an estimate of casualty totals under standards prevailing since 1984. See notes.

2 Number of casualties: by county, by type of road user: 1993

	Children (0-15)	Adults (16-59)	Elderly (60+)	All[1] casualties	Pedest-rians	Pedal cyclists	Motor cyclists	'Car occupants	Other[2] road users
Avon	463	2,704	382	3,577	599	340	449	1,993	196
Bedfordshire	367	2,193	229	2,789	351	198	217	1,832	191
Berkshire	426	2,760	304	3,668	454	333	307	2,407	167
Buckinghamshire	442	2,792	275	3,670	323	243	306	2,580	218
Cambridgeshire	507	3,489	416	4,462	319	744	419	2,735	245
Cheshire	645	4,489	578	5,712	617	403	393	3,915	384
Cleveland	502	1,830	215	2,547	529	211	102	1,538	167
Cornwall	353	1,891	352	2,604	344	174	289	1,631	166
Cumbria	389	1,926	303	2,618	358	185	209	1,688	178
Derbyshire	708	3,640	477	5,004	645	330	487	3,267	275
Devon	638	3,703	675	5,023	767	395	599	3,055	207
Dorset	378	2,504	536	3,418	331	327	372	2,199	189
Durham	512	2,069	246	2,827	412	159	125	1,863	268
East Sussex	451	2,596	570	3,617	576	272	314	2,161	294
Essex	991	6,299	885	8,648	923	647	704	5,869	505
Gloucestershire	327	2,134	291	2,752	314	254	266	1,764	154
Greater London	5,372	33,058	4,578	45,927	9,709	4,198	5,532	22,511	3,977
Greater Manchester	2,705	11,947	1,540	16,192	3,270	1,261	762	9,900	999
Hampshire	1,066	6,798	923	8,787	967	983	939	5,465	433
Hereford & Worcester	386	2,471	383	3,240	331	317	321	2,113	158
Hertfordshire	715	4,522	561	5,853	582	392	503	4,070	306
Humberside	793	3,223	514	4,737	742	694	518	2,364	419
Isle of Wight	86	378	85	549	80	35	67	335	32
Kent	1,105	6,021	852	8,068	1,079	561	857	5,065	506
Lancashire	1,283	5,916	937	8,169	1,326	603	546	5,153	541
Leicestershire	653	3,522	441	4,679	660	423	356	2,942	298
Lincolnshire	501	2,692	493	3,686	300	316	292	2,493	285
Merseyside	1,692	7,653	1,092	10,437	1,751	632	357	6,959	738
Norfolk	558	3,375	632	4,713	454	405	482	3,150	222
Northamptonshire	420	2,328	288	3,042	370	204	253	2,082	133
Northumberland	191	1,162	193	1,546	163	87	64	1,093	139
North Yorkshire	492	3,419	595	4,528	436	334	458	3,013	287
Nottinghamshire	852	4,042	572	5,796	897	479	506	3,472	442
Oxfordshire	322	2,291	320	3,122	268	342	277	2,072	163
Shropshire	240	1,686	246	2,172	181	165	167	1,563	96
Somerset	259	1,493	251	2,155	223	149	185	1,449	149
South Yorkshire	962	4,339	702	6,003	1,086	392	333	3,541	651
Staffordshire	814	4,995	553	6,362	756	426	444	4,350	386
Suffolk	351	2,297	392	3,045	303	275	373	1,947	147
Surrey	685	5,384	742	6,985	589	558	640	4,824	374
Tyne & Wear	853	2,987	502	4,342	1,112	302	162	2,339	427
Warwickshire	339	2,341	264	3,082	281	226	277	2,084	214
West Midlands	2,223	8,254	1,266	11,743	2,675	875	699	6,816	678
West Sussex	404	2,566	459	3,429	316	375	321	2,219	198
West Yorkshire	1,766	7,805	1,192	10,763	2,147	631	545	6,570	870
Wiltshire	384	2,479	335	3,199	287	245	317	2,135	215
England	36,571	198,463	28,637	269,287	41,203	22,100	23,111	164,586	18,287
Wales	2,334	10,314	1,677	14,331	2,182	777	850	9,573	949
Scotland	3,685	15,990	2,713	22,402	4,713	1,191	1,105	13,298	2,095
Great Britain	42,590	224,767	33,027	306,020	48,098	24,068	25,066	187,457	21,331
Northern Ireland	1,571	8,633	896	11,100	1,275	282	250	8,277	1,016
United Kingdom	44,161	233,400	33,923	317,120	49,373	24,350	25,316	195,734	22,347

Number of casualties

1 Includes age not reported.
2 Includes road user type not known.

3 Number of casualties: by county, by type of road user: 1981-85 average[1]

	Children (0-15)	Adults (16-59)	Older adults (60+)	All[2] casualties	Pedest-rians	Pedal cyclists	Motor cyclists	Car occupants	Other[3] road users
Avon	616	3,520	447	4,584	777	402	1,399	1,768	238
Bedfordshire	502	2,480	252	3,235	495	299	628	1,552	262
Berkshire	573	3,232	333	4,243	567	449	904	2,167	157
Buckinghamshire	464	2,713	283	3,504	409	287	700	1,940	168
Cambridgeshire	489	3,095	397	3,981	345	646	923	1,834	233
Cheshire	803	3,789	490	5,095	711	593	1,126	2,324	341
Cleveland	587	1,853	231	2,671	682	274	515	1,016	185
Cornwall	359	2,079	253	2,691	339	151	756	1,301	144
Cumbria	441	2,068	297	2,806	444	216	606	1,383	157
Derbyshire	715	3,505	439	4,933	808	405	1,207	2,098	415
Devon	769	4,333	624	5,726	845	400	1,654	2,526	302
Dorset	461	2,745	471	3,677	487	396	959	1,647	188
Durham	450	1,806	221	2,476	510	140	412	1,216	198
East Sussex	535	2,722	655	3,911	725	287	830	1,842	227
Essex	1,344	7,165	947	9,474	1,212	803	1,845	5,003	611
Gloucestershire	419	2,549	308	3,276	378	348	926	1,465	160
Greater London	7,106	37,831	5,855	54,156	13,081	4,739	9,957	21,778	4,601
Greater Manchester	2,946	9,320	1,431	13,699	3,931	1,376	2,284	5,186	922
Hampshire	1,276	7,151	881	9,308	1,159	1,182	2,530	3,981	456
Hereford & Worcester	491	2,895	384	3,770	461	370	847	1,909	183
Hertfordshire	784	4,401	485	5,729	738	511	1,173	3,003	304
Humberside	842	3,601	491	4,934	821	727	1,377	1,620	388
Isle of Wight	107	481	74	662	107	61	206	260	28
Kent	1,251	6,769	848	8,867	1,246	744	2,291	4,139	447
Lancashire	1,399	5,155	906	7,460	1,683	666	1,458	3,188	466
Leicestershire	752	3,657	415	4,825	827	507	1,117	2,124	249
Lincolnshire	501	2,866	382	3,749	365	381	852	1,929	221
Merseyside	1,632	4,718	875	7,225	2,066	583	1,009	2,926	642
Norfolk	551	3,195	495	4,241	483	456	1,063	1,999	240
Northamptonshire	499	2,818	334	3,652	449	240	779	1,913	271
Northumberland	215	1,142	159	1,516	192	95	270	828	131
North Yorkshire	568	3,349	496	4,413	531	420	1,030	2,150	283
Nottinghamshire	987	4,364	570	5,920	1,111	609	1,362	2,381	458
Oxfordshire	389	2,677	297	3,424	362	382	798	1,663	219
Shropshire	297	1,767	211	2,275	252	185	473	1,237	129
Somerset	299	1,875	276	2,450	267	222	640	1,204	117
South Yorkshire	1,108	4,121	685	5,914	1,475	354	1,069	2,308	708
Staffordshire	1,038	4,972	518	6,528	983	558	1,388	3,167	432
Suffolk	479	2,762	385	3,627	397	389	961	1,696	183
Surrey	921	5,844	779	7,640	808	838	1,764	3,918	312
Tyne & Wear	1,028	2,906	509	4,443	1,491	334	650	1,568	400
Warwickshire	400	2,179	261	2,839	339	295	606	1,446	154
West Midlands	2,714	8,345	1,227	12,286	3,596	1,064	1,993	4,812	820
West Sussex	498	2,919	527	3,943	440	464	907	1,953	180
West Yorkshire	2,039	7,531	1,084	10,654	2,728	722	2,048	4,386	770
Wiltshire	491	3,080	377	3,948	392	358	887	2,056	256
England	43,133	204,343	28,867	280,382	52,515	25,927	59,179	123,806	18,956
Wales	2,320	10,500	1,576	14,395	2,666	857	2,566	7,211	1,094
Scotland	4,881	19,157	3,097	27,134	6,560	1,607	3,446	12,924	2,598
Great Britain	50,334	234,000	33,540	321,912	61,741	28,391	65,191	143,941	22,647
Northern Ireland[4]	1,516	5,954	731	8,204	1,648	399	765	5,398	
United Kingdom[4]	51,850	239,954	34,271	330,115	63,389	28,791	65,956	171,986	

1 Figures have been rounded so there may be an apparent slight discrepancy between the sum of the constituent items and the total as shown.
2 Includes age not reported.
3 Includes road user type not known.
4 It is not possible to give separate casualty figures for car occupants and other road users for Northern Ireland for these years.

4 Total casualty rates[1] : by county, by type of road user: 1993

Rate per 100,000 population

	Children (0-15)	Adults (16-59)	Elderly (60+)	All[2] casualties	Pedest- rians	Pedal cyclists	Motor cyclists	Car occupants	Other[3] road users
Avon	248	470	185	369	62	35	46	206	20
Bedfordshire	306	672	253	520	65	37	40	341	36
Berkshire	265	586	241	484	60	44	40	318	22
Buckinghamshire	311	706	255	568	50	38	47	400	34
Cambridgeshire	365	846	330	658	47	110	62	404	36
Cheshire	320	784	300	591	64	42	41	405	40
Cleveland	396	561	201	455	94	38	18	275	30
Cornwall	386	720	291	548	72	37	61	343	35
Cumbria	409	682	269	534	73	38	43	344	36
Derbyshire	376	654	236	528	68	35	51	345	29
Devon	328	633	254	481	73	38	57	292	20
Dorset	322	696	287	515	50	49	56	331	28
Durham	417	582	191	466	68	26	21	307	44
East Sussex	353	662	284	502	80	38	44	300	41
Essex	316	689	270	556	59	42	45	377	32
Gloucestershire	305	680	241	508	58	47	49	326	28
Greater London	393	773	362	665	141	61	80	326	58
Greater Manchester	488	791	302	629	127	49	30	385	39
Hampshire	334	716	290	554	61	62	59	344	27
Hereford & Worcester	275	614	259	469	48	46	46	306	23
Hertfordshire	351	758	289	589	59	39	51	409	31
Humberside	432	630	276	537	84	79	59	268	48
Isle of Wight	375	573	232	437	64	28	53	267	25
Kent	351	674	258	524	70	36	56	329	33
Lancashire	436	731	302	578	94	43	39	365	38
Leicestershire	344	655	252	519	73	47	39	326	33
Lincolnshire	437	793	345	618	50	53	49	418	48
Merseyside	552	920	355	722	121	44	25	481	51
Norfolk	393	780	336	618	60	53	63	413	29
Northamptonshire	307	664	259	515	63	35	43	353	23
Northumberland	312	655	282	503	53	28	21	356	45
North Yorkshire	360	813	359	626	60	46	63	417	40
Nottinghamshire	413	664	272	565	87	47	49	339	43
Oxfordshire	269	634	301	532	46	58	47	353	28
Shropshire	282	696	288	526	44	40	40	379	23
Somerset	277	567	217	456	47	32	39	307	32
South Yorkshire	371	562	256	460	83	30	26	271	50
Staffordshire	379	792	268	605	72	41	42	414	37
Suffolk	264	624	267	470	47	42	58	300	23
Surrey	345	872	337	674	57	54	62	465	36
Tyne & Wear	373	451	206	383	98	27	14	206	38
Warwickshire	348	799	260	626	57	46	56	424	44
West Midlands	392	540	237	446	102	33	27	259	26
West Sussex	302	656	245	481	44	53	45	311	28
West Yorkshire	397	632	288	514	103	30	26	314	42
Wiltshire	323	720	289	552	50	42	55	369	37
England	373	696	285	557	85	46	48	340	38
Wales	81	625	257	494	75	27	29	330	33
Scotland	359	524	262	438	92	23	22	260	41
Great Britain	373	677	282	543	85	43	44	332	38
Northern Ireland	379	936	328	689	79	18	16	514	63
United Kingdom	374	684	283	547	85	42	44	337	38

1 Based on final 1992 population estimates.
2 Includes age not reported.
3 Includes road user type not known.

5 Casualty indicators: by county, by type of road user: 1993

	Children[1] (0-15)	Adults[1] (16-59)	Elderly[1] (60+)	Pedestrians	Pedal cyclists	Motor cyclists	Car occupants	Other[2] road users
	Percentage of all casualties who are:						Percentage of all casualties	
Avon	13.0	76.2	10.8	16.7	9.5	12.6	55.7	5.5
Bedfordshire	13.2	78.6	8.2	12.6	7.1	7.8	65.7	6.8
Berkshire	12.2	79.1	8.7	12.4	9.1	8.4	65.6	4.6
Buckinghamshire	12.6	79.6	7.8	8.8	6.6	8.3	70.3	5.9
Cambridgeshire	11.5	79.1	9.4	7.1	16.7	9.4	61.3	5.5
Cheshire	11.3	78.6	10.1	10.8	7.1	6.9	68.5	6.7
Cleveland	19.7	71.8	8.4	20.8	8.3	4.0	60.4	6.6
Cornwall	13.6	72.8	13.6	13.2	6.7	11.1	62.6	6.4
Cumbria	14.9	73.6	11.6	13.7	7.1	8.0	64.5	6.8
Derbyshire	14.7	75.4	9.9	12.9	6.6	9.7	65.3	5.5
Devon	12.7	73.8	13.5	15.3	7.9	11.9	60.8	4.1
Dorset	11.1	73.3	15.7	9.7	9.6	10.9	64.3	5.5
Durham	18.1	73.2	8.7	14.6	5.6	4.4	65.9	9.5
East Sussex	12.5	71.8	15.8	15.9	7.5	8.7	59.7	8.1
Essex	12.1	77.1	10.8	10.7	7.5	8.1	67.9	5.8
Gloucestershire	11.9	77.5	10.6	11.4	9.2	9.7	64.1	5.6
Greater London	12.5	76.9	10.6	21.1	9.1	12.0	49.0	8.7
Greater Manchester	16.7	73.8	9.5	20.2	7.8	4.7	61.1	6.2
Hampshire	12.1	77.4	10.5	11.0	11.2	10.7	62.2	4.9
Hereford & Worcester	11.9	76.3	11.8	10.2	9.8	9.9	65.2	4.9
Hertfordshire	12.3	78.0	9.7	9.9	6.7	8.6	69.5	5.2
Humberside	17.5	71.1	11.3	15.7	14.7	10.9	49.9	8.8
Isle of Wight	15.7	68.9	15.5	14.6	6.4	12.2	61.0	5.8
Kent	13.9	75.5	10.7	13.4	7.0	10.6	62.8	6.3
Lancashire	15.8	72.7	11.5	16.2	7.4	6.7	63.1	6.6
Leicestershire	14.1	76.3	9.6	14.1	9.0	7.6	62.9	6.4
Lincolnshire	13.6	73.0	13.4	8.1	8.6	7.9	67.6	7.7
Merseyside	16.2	73.3	10.5	16.8	6.1	3.4	66.7	7.1
Norfolk	12.2	73.9	13.8	9.6	8.6	10.2	66.8	4.7
Northamptonshire	13.8	76.7	9.5	12.2	6.7	8.3	68.4	4.4
Northumberland	12.4	75.2	12.5	10.5	5.6	4.1	70.7	9.0
North Yorkshire	10.9	75.9	13.2	9.6	7.4	10.1	66.5	6.3
Nottinghamshire	15.6	73.9	10.5	15.5	8.3	8.7	59.9	7.6
Oxfordshire	11.0	78.1	10.9	8.6	11.0	8.9	66.4	5.2
Shropshire	11.0	77.6	11.3	8.3	7.6	7.7	72.0	4.4
Somerset	12.9	74.5	12.5	10.3	6.9	8.6	67.2	6.9
South Yorkshire	16.0	72.3	11.7	18.1	6.5	5.5	59.0	10.8
Staffordshire	12.8	78.5	8.7	11.9	6.7	7.0	68.4	6.1
Suffolk	11.5	75.6	12.9	10.0	9.0	12.2	63.9	4.8
Surrey	10.1	79.0	10.9	8.4	8.0	9.2	69.1	5.4
Tyne & Wear	19.6	68.8	11.6	25.6	7.0	3.7	53.9	9.8
Warwickshire	11.5	79.5	9.0	9.1	7.3	9.0	67.6	6.9
West Midlands	18.9	70.3	10.8	22.8	7.5	6.0	58.0	5.8
West Sussex	11.8	74.8	13.4	9.2	10.9	9.4	64.7	5.8
West Yorkshire	16.4	72.5	11.1	19.9	5.9	5.1	61.0	8.1
Wiltshire	12.0	77.5	10.5	9.0	7.7	9.9	66.7	6.7
England	13.9	75.3	10.9	15.3	8.2	8.6	61.1	6.8
Wales	16.3	72.0	11.7	15.2	5.4	5.9	66.8	6.6
Scotland	16.5	71.4	12.1	21.0	5.3	4.9	59.4	9.4
Great Britain	14.2	74.8	11.0	15.7	7.9	8.2	61.3	7.0
Northern Ireland	14.2	77.8	8.1	11.5	2.5	2.3	74.6	9.2
United Kingdom	13.9	73.6	10.7	15.6	7.7	8.0	61.7	7.0

1 Percentage of casualties of known age.
2 Includes road user type not known.

25

6 Casualty changes: by county and severity: 1981-85 average, 1993

	Fatal and serious casualties			Total casualties		Number of casualties
	1981-85 average	1993	percentage change	1981-85 average	1993	percentage change
Avon	1,356	554	-59.2	4,584	3,577	-22.0
Bedfordshire	714	417	-41.6	3,235	2,789	-13.8
Berkshire	1,095	379	-65.4	4,243	3,668	-13.6
Buckinghamshire	1,031	414	-59.8	3,504	3,670	4.7
Cambridgeshire	1,087	855	-21.3	3,981	4,462	12.1
Cheshire	916	612	-33.2	5,095	5,712	12.1
Cleveland	486	361	-25.8	2,671	2,547	-4.7
Cornwall	858	429	-50.0	2,691	2,604	-3.2
Cumbria	829	488	-41.1	2,806	2,618	-6.7
Derbyshire	1,222	572	-53.2	4,933	5,004	1.4
Devon	1,897	933	-50.8	5,726	5,023	-12.3
Dorset	940	513	-45.4	3,677	3,418	-7.0
Durham	703	329	-53.2	2,476	2,827	14.2
East Sussex	989	592	-40.1	3,911	3,617	-7.5
Essex	2,398	1,327	-44.7	9,474	8,648	-8.7
Gloucestershire	1,166	465	-60.1	3,276	2,752	-16.0
Greater London[1]	8,230 (9,175)	6,419	-22.0	54,156	45,927	-15.2
Greater Manchester	2,362	1,605	-32.0	13,699	16,192	18.2
Hampshire	2,755	1,474	-46.5	9,308	8,787	-5.6
Hereford & Worcester	1,071	527	-50.8	3,770	3,240	-14.1
Hertfordshire	1,388	1,038	-25.2	5,729	5,853	2.2
Humberside	1,129	970	-14.1	4,934	4,737	-4.0
Isle of Wight	184	102	-44.6	662	549	-17.0
Kent	2,385	1,397	-41.4	8,867	8,068	-9.0
Lancashire	1,704	1,490	-12.6	7,460	8,169	9.5
Leicestershire	1,226	644	-47.5	4,825	4,679	-3.0
Lincolnshire	1,074	829	-22.8	3,749	3,686	-1.7
Merseyside	1,237	998	-19.3	7,225	10,437	44.4
Norfolk	1,524	998	-34.5	4,241	4,713	11.1
Northamptonshire	1,328	723	-45.5	3,652	3,042	-16.7
Northumberland	400	287	-28.2	1,516	1,546	2.0
North Yorkshire	1,835	1,323	-27.9	4,413	4,528	2.6
Nottinghamshire	1,540	1,172	-23.9	5,920	5,796	-2.1
Oxfordshire	1,067	410	-61.6	3,424	3,122	-8.8
Shropshire	833	472	-43.3	2,275	2,172	-4.5
Somerset	811	392	-51.6	2,450	2,155	-12.0
South Yorkshire	1,320	696	-47.3	5,914	6,003	1.5
Staffordshire	1,442	650	-54.9	6,528	6,362	-2.5
Suffolk	1,170	607	-48.1	3,627	3,045	-16.0
Surrey	1,641	980	-40.3	7,640	6,985	-8.6
Tyne & Wear	1,048	713	-32.0	4,443	4,342	-2.3
Warwickshire	1,059	745	-29.7	2,839	3,082	8.5
West Midlands	3,452	2,120	-38.6	12,286	11,743	-4.4
West Sussex	922	525	-43.0	3,943	3,429	-13.0
West Yorkshire	2,547	1,614	-36.6	10,654	10,763	1.0
Wiltshire	1,019	630	-38.2	3,948	3,199	-19.0
England	67,388	41,790	-38.0	280,382	269,287	-4.0
Wales	3,855	2,189	-43.2	14,395	14,331	-0.4
Scotland	8,887	4,844	-45.5	27,134	22,402	-17.4
Great Britain	80,130	48,823	-39.1	321,912	306,020	-4.9
Northern Ireland	2,362	1,868	-20.9	8,204	11,100	35.3
United Kingdom	82,492	50,691	-38.6	330,115	317,120	-3.9

1 In September 1984 the Metropolitan Police implemented revised standards in the assessment of serious casualties.
  Figures in brackets estimate casualty totals under standards prevailing since 1984. See preface.

7 Number of casualties: by road class, region[1] and severity: 1993

Number of casualties

	Motorways	Built up				Non built up				All roads[2]
		Trunk	Principal	Other	Total	Trunk	Principal	Other	Total	
Northern[3]										
Killed	11	0	39	67	106	52	37	24	113	230
Killed or Seriously Injured	47	28	406	881	1,315	244	318	254	816	2,178
All Casualties	337	230	2,844	5,797	8,871	1,418	1,809	1,445	4,672	13,880
Yorkshire and Humberside										
Killed	17	11	96	94	201	38	77	54	169	387
Killed or Seriously Injured	96	87	1,032	1,707	2,826	375	681	625	1,681	4,603
All Casualties	810	628	6,942	11,239	18,809	1,429	2,577	2,406	6,412	26,031
East Midlands										
Killed	12	15	44	48	107	73	83	75	231	350
Killed or Seriously Injured	120	124	626	1,148	1,898	467	750	705	1,922	3,940
All Casualties	778	865	4,285	7,597	12,747	2,186	3,367	3,129	8,682	22,207
Eastern										
Killed	26	2	53	69	124	96	115	94	305	455
Killed or Seriously Injured	230	60	795	1,660	2,515	681	1,047	1,183	2,911	5,656
All Casualties	1,713	545	5,937	11,015	17,497	3,111	4,985	5,873	13,969	33,180
South East										
Killed	31	11	89	91	191	54	116	86	256	478[1]
Killed or Seriously Injured	315	82	1,262	1,832	3,176	387	1,025	955	2,367	5,859
All Casualties	2,250	638	9,107	13,150	22,895	2,223	5,601	5,248	13,072	38,225
London										
Killed	3	35	141	90	266	15	2	0	17	286
Killed or Seriously Injured	73	589	3,188	2,319	6,096	181	33	35	249	6,419
All Casualties	634	4,355	22,835	16,673	43,863	1,039	208	181	1,428	45,927
South West										
Killed	15	2	38	54	94	46	102	52	200	310
Killed or Seriously Injured	94	36	599	1,218	1,853	312	852	795	1,959	3,916
All Casualties	628	297	4,120	7,824	12,241	1,667	4,214	3,934	9,815	22,728
West Midlands										
Killed	39	5	80	80	165	47	65	37	149	353
Killed or Seriously Injured	251	69	1,123	1,759	2,951	367	466	479	1,312	4,514
All Casualties	1,304	645	7,341	10,813	18,799	1,609	2,417	2,470	6,496	26,599
North West[3]										
Killed	27	5	138	112	255	19	59	19	97	379
Killed or Seriously Injured	188	73	1,532	2,017	3,622	217	363	312	892	4,705
All Casualties	1,872	879	14,373	17,915	33,167	1,327	2,345	1,787	5,459	40,510
England										
Killed	181	86	718	705	1,509	440	656	441	1,537	3,228
Killed or Seriously Injured	1,414	1,148	10,563	14,541	26,252	3,231	5,535	5,343	14,109	41,790
All Casualties	10,326	9,082	77,784	102,023	188,889	16,009	27,523	26,473	70,005	269,287
Wales										
Killed	2	5	26	46	77	51	40	17	108	187
Killed or Seriously Injured	20	72	357	634	1,063	405	380	321	1,106	2,189
All Casualties	233	531	2,833	5,391	8,755	1,827	1,832	1,684	5,343	14,331
Scotland										
Killed	18	9	52	73	134	98	97	52	247	399
Killed or Seriously Injured	105	130	759	1,567	2,456	738	866	679	2,283	4,844
All Casualties	487	588	4,404	8,359	13,351	2,620	3,244	2,700	8,564	22,402
Great Britain										
Killed	201	100	796	824	1,720	589	793	510	1,892	3,814
Killed or Seriously Injured	1,539	1,350	11,679	16,742	29,771	4,374	6,781	6,343	17,498	48,823
All Casualties	11,046	10,201	85,021	115,773	210,995	20,456	32,599	30,857	83,912	306,020

1 Casualty data by road class are not available for Northern Ireland.
2 Includes speed limit not reported.
3 From 1st April 1991 responsibilty for Cumbria transferred from the North West Regional Office to the Northern Regional Office.
The change to the road accident database was deferred until 1992. Consequently data prior to 1992 for both Northern and North West regions shown in this table in previous editions of RASER are not comparable with the 1993 data presented above.

8 Casualty rates per 100 million vehicle kilometres: by road class, region[1] and severity: 1991-1993 average

Rate per 100 million vehicle kilometres[2]

		A roads				All A roads	All major roads[3]
		Built up		Non built up			
	Motorways	Trunk	Principal	Trunk	Principal		
Northern[4]							
Fatal	0.8	1.4	1.3	1.5	1.5	1.4	1.3
Fatal or serious	3.2	19.2	16.2	7.9	10.4	11.3	10.2
All severities	19.8	128.7	109.2	41.9	52.7	65.8	59.7
Yorkshire and Humberside							
Fatal	0.4	1.7	1.4	1.0	2.0	1.5	1.2
Fatal or serious	2.7	14.7	17.5	9.5	17.5	15.1	12.1
All severities	16.8	89.5	107.0	34.7	64.5	74.2	60.6
East Midlands							
Fatal	0.4	1.4	1.3	1.3	1.7	1.5	1.3
Fatal or serious	3.4	15.2	17.0	8.2	15.3	13.0	11.2
All severities	19.3	98.7	114.5	36.8	66.4	68.6	59.1
Eastern							
Fatal	0.3	0.9	1.0	0.9	1.4	1.1	0.9
Fatal or serious	2.6	14.1	15.0	6.8	11.5	10.5	8.5
All severities	17.6	89.7	101.7	30.9	52.8	56.1	46.2
South East							
Fatal	0.3	1.5	0.9	0.7	1.1	0.9	0.7
Fatal or serious	2.3	16.8	13.8	4.7	10.4	10.0	7.6
All severities	15.7	112.3	97.1	27.1	52.8	60.7	46.7
London							
Fatal	0.3	1.4	1.5	0.5	1.0	1.3	1.2
Fatal or serious	6.1	21.1	32.5	5.7	11.2	25.3	23.9
All severities	50.3	142.5	211.5	32.6	62.5	164.3	156.5
South West							
Fatal	0.3	0.8	0.9	1.0	1.4	1.1	1.0
Fatal or serious	1.9	11.7	11.5	6.4	11.3	10.0	8.3
All severities	11.6	90.9	72.4	30.3	50.3	52.0	43.5
West Midlands							
Fatal	0.4	1.3	1.3	1.2	1.4	1.3	1.0
Fatal or serious	2.6	12.5	17.4	9.8	11.6	13.7	10.0
All severities	15.4	85.9	106.5	41.8	54.7	75.4	55.4
North West[4]							
Fatal	0.4	1.3	1.4	0.9	1.4	1.3	1.0
Fatal or serious	2.1	11.6	15.3	7.0	9.6	12.5	8.8
All severities	18.7	125.7	136.5	43.3	57.2	102.8	73.2
England							
Fatal	0.4	1.3	1.2	1.0	1.4	1.2	1.0
Fatal or serious	2.5	16.8	18.3	7.1	11.9	13.1	10.4
All severities	17.3	116.4	125.4	33.8	55.3	77.9	62.6
Wales							
Fatal	0.2	0.9	1.2	1.2	1.3	1.2	1.1
Fatal or serious	1.7	11.9	13.5	10.7	12.9	12.2	10.7
All severities	14.8	76.2	99.1	44.5	59.7	65.6	58.5
Scotland							
Fatal	0.6	1.4	1.2	1.6	1.6	1.5	1.4
Fatal or serious	3.2	20.4	18.6	11.9	15.4	15.1	13.4
All severities	14.6	90.4	94.9	39.7	55.0	61.5	54.5
Great Britain							
Fatal	0.4	1.3	1.2	1.1	1.5	1.3	1.0
Fatal or serious	2.6	16.7	18.1	7.9	12.3	13.2	10.7
All severities	17.1	111.3	122.0	35.3	55.5	75.6	61.7

1 Traffic data and casualty data in this breakdown are not available for Northern Ireland.
2 Traffic for 1992 has been revised.
3 Includes road class and type not reported.
4 From 1st April 1991 responsibilty for Cumbria transferred from the North West Regional Office to the Northern Regional Office.
   The change to the road accident database was deferred until 1992.

9 Accident rates per 100 million vehicle kilometres: by road class, region[1] and severity: 1991-1993 average

Rate per 100 million vehicle kilometres[2]

	Motorways	A roads Built up Trunk	A roads Built up Principal	A roads Non built up Trunk	A roads Non built up Principal	All A roads	All major roads[3]
Northern[4]							
Fatal	0.6	1.4	1.3	1.3	1.2	1.3	1.2
Fatal or serious	2.4	17.6	14.9	5.6	7.7	9.1	8.2
All severities	12.1	94.7	83.9	24.7	32.3	45.0	40.6
Yorkshire and Humberside							
Fatal	0.4	1.4	1.3	0.9	1.7	1.3	1.1
Fatal or serious	2.0	12.1	15.5	6.7	12.2	11.9	9.6
All severities	10.5	67.4	82.2	20.4	39.0	52.5	42.5
East Midlands							
Fatal	0.4	1.3	1.3	1.1	1.5	1.3	1.1
Fatal or serious	2.2	13.7	15.3	6.1	11.1	10.4	8.8
All severities	10.8	74.9	89.0	22.1	40.8	47.2	40.2
Eastern							
Fatal	0.3	0.8	0.9	0.8	1.3	1.0	0.8
Fatal or serious	2.0	12.1	13.5	4.9	8.5	8.3	6.7
All severities	11.1	69.5	79.4	19.0	33.6	39.0	31.9
South East							
Fatal	0.2	1.4	0.8	0.6	1.0	0.9	0.7
Fatal or serious	1.7	14.0	12.7	3.7	7.9	8.3	6.3
All severities	9.6	84.7	77.4	17.3	34.5	44.2	33.5
London							
Fatal	0.2	1.3	1.4	0.4	1.0	1.2	1.1
Fatal or serious	4.7	18.4	30.0	4.8	9.0	23.0	21.8
All severities	35.6	114.5	180.1	23.7	44.9	137.7	130.7
South West							
Fatal	0.2	0.8	0.8	0.8	1.2	1.0	0.8
Fatal or serious	1.4	10.0	10.3	4.6	8.5	8.0	6.6
All severities	7.5	70.5	58.0	18.5	32.1	36.6	30.4
West Midlands							
Fatal	0.2	1.3	1.3	1.0	1.2	1.2	0.9
Fatal or serious	1.8	10.7	15.2	6.9	8.7	11.2	8.1
All severities	9.3	63.3	81.7	26.6	35.0	54.5	39.4
North West[4]							
Fatal	0.3	1.2	1.4	0.8	1.2	1.2	0.9
Fatal or serious	1.6	10.1	13.9	5.2	7.2	10.8	7.6
All severities	11.8	89.1	100.3	26.3	35.8	73.1	51.5
England							
Fatal	0.3	1.3	1.2	0.8	1.3	1.1	0.9
Fatal or serious	1.9	14.6	16.6	5.2	8.8	10.9	8.6
All severities	10.8	90.1	99.4	21.0	35.0	57.3	45.6
Wales							
Fatal	0.1	0.9	1.1	1.0	1.1	1.1	0.9
Fatal or serious	1.3	9.9	11.4	7.3	9.4	9.2	8.1
All severities	9.3	55.0	72.1	25.3	36.4	43.0	38.3
Scotland							
Fatal	0.5	1.4	1.1	1.4	1.4	1.3	1.2
Fatal or serious	2.5	17.5	17.2	8.2	11.2	12.0	10.5
All severities	9.4	67.7	77.0	23.6	34.6	43.3	38.2
Great Britain							
Fatal	0.3	1.2	1.2	0.9	1.3	1.1	0.9
Fatal or serious	1.9	14.5	16.4	5.7	9.1	10.9	8.8
All severities	10.7	85.7	96.6	21.6	35.1	55.2	44.6

1 Traffic data and casualty data in this breakdown are not available for Northern Ireland.

2 Traffic for 1992 has been revised.

3 Includes road class and type not reported.

4 From 1st April 1991 responsibilty for Cumbria transferred from the North West Regional Office to the Northern Regional Office. This change to road accident database was deferred until 1992. Consequently data prior to 1992 for both Northern and North West regions shown in this table in previous editions of RASER are not comparable with the 1993 data presented above.

10 Accident indices[1]: by month, severity and region: accidents by severity and region: 1993

	Jan	Feb	Mar	Apr	May	Jun	Jul	Aug	Sep	Oct	Nov	Dec	Index/number All accidents
Northern[2]													
Fatal & serious	99	100	84	105	110	98	109	87	102	102	91	112	1,876
All	91	93	84	97	96	102	111	94	106	104	110	113	9,936
Yorkshire and Humberside													
Fatal & serious	91	106	84	95	99	114	99	101	99	93	109	112	3,810
All	91	90	89	91	100	98	106	97	107	102	118	110	19,276
East Midlands													
Fatal & serious	93	92	89	100	100	100	86	100	106	115	104	114	3,289
All	93	91	86	96	97	99	101	95	107	111	111	113	15,850
Eastern													
Fatal & serious	94	87	83	85	103	99	107	95	101	114	115	116	4,697
All	93	87	89	91	98	102	109	91	106	107	117	109	24,016
South East													
Fatal & serious	92	81	99	94	92	101	102	95	111	106	110	115	5,010
All	98	82	93	94	99	102	105	93	108	106	115	104	28,371
London													
Fatal & serious	98	101	99	94	109	105	95	92	98	106	104	101	5,842
All	92	89	97	99	102	105	102	92	109	105	109	100	38,533
South West													
Fatal & serious	85	82	91	97	102	107	110	101	118	96	109	103	3,290
All	88	81	89	98	103	104	110	103	110	98	106	108	17,014
West Midlands													
Fatal & serious	90	80	94	106	110	100	107	94	111	99	103	106	3,769
All	94	90	87	97	109	99	107	88	107	102	109	112	19,783
North West[2]													
Fatal & serious	97	73	90	102	103	105	96	99	103	109	103	118	4,168
All	97	84	95	98	105	100	100	97	101	102	110	109	29,363
England													
Fatal & serious	93	89	91	97	103	103	100	96	105	105	106	111	35,751
All	93	87	91	96	101	102	105	94	106	104	112	108	202,142
Wales[2]													
Fatal & serious	87	80	83	89	121	94	123	108	112	91	104	106	1,747
All	86	80	84	104	108	101	112	107	111	96	99	111	10,049
Scotland													
Fatal & serious	103	94	87	84	95	96	104	105	102	96	108	125	4,003
All	94	92	94	98	100	98	99	104	109	92	103	116	16,674
Great Britain													
Fatal & serious	94	89	91	95	103	102	102	97	105	103	107	112	41,501
All	93	87	91	96	102	102	105	95	107	103	110	108	228,865
Northern Ireland													
Fatal & serious	93	114	103	85	101	115	98	89	111	89	94	109	1,378
All	98	109	97	91	102	97	100	87	111	89	104	116	6,517
United Kingdom													
Fatal & serious	94	90	91	95	103	103	102	97	105	103	106	112	42,879
All	93	88	91	96	102	101	104	95	107	102	110	109	235,382

1 The base(=100) is the average number of accidents per day for the region.
2 From 1st April 1991 responsibilty for Cumbria transferred from the North West Regional Office to the Northern Regional Office.
   The change to the road accident database was deferred until 1992. Consequently data prior to 1992 for both Northern and North West regions shown in
   this table in previous editions of RASER are not comparable with the 1993 data presented above.

11 Accidents on motorways: by carriageway type, junction, number of lanes, region[1] and severity: 1993

Number of accidents

	Junction			Non-junction		
	Number of lanes		Circular section of roundabouts	Number of lanes		Total[2]
	2	3+		2	3+	
Northern[3]						
Fatal or serious	0	3	1	11	18	36
All severities	18	9	16	60	68	186
Yorkshire and Humberside						
Fatal or serious	6	5	3	11	50	77
All severities	32	23	78	70	277	518
East Midlands						
Fatal or serious	1	12	1	3	66	87
All severities	7	35	19	10	351	450
Eastern						
Fatal or serious	4	12	2	25	125	177
All severities	25	75	6	132	745	1,059
South East						
Fatal or serious	7	14	4	27	159	234
All severities	64	64	63	180	869	1,373
London						
Fatal or serious	4	4	0	14	39	61
All severities	44	67	8	66	236	435
of which:						
Inner London						
Fatal or serious	0	0	0	2	1	3
All severities	9	4	6	6	7	39
Outer London						
Fatal or serious	4	4	0	12	38	58
All severities	35	63	2	60	229	396
South West						
Fatal or serious	1	3	0	5	50	68
All severities	13	30	23	33	275	409
West Midlands						
Fatal or serious	1	11	1	14	122	160
All severities	7	59	15	56	595	788
North West[3]						
Fatal or serious	4	6	2	13	106	147
All severities	70	75	67	107	732	1,209
England						
Fatal or serious	28	70	14	123	735	1,047
All severities	280	437	295	714	4,148	6,427
Wales						
Fatal or serious	0	1	0	5	11	17
All severities	4	4	8	65	69	153
Scotland						
Fatal or serious	8	5	0	33	19	74
All severities	27	13	1	119	89	283
Great Britain						
Fatal or serious	36	76	14	161	765	1,138
All severities	311	454	304	898	4,306	6,863

1 Accident data are not available in this breakdown for Northern Ireland.

2 Includes unknown carriageway type and slip roads.

3 From 1st April 1991 responsibilty for Cumbria transferred from the North West Regional Office to the Northern Regional Office.
   The change to the road accident database was deferred until 1992. Consequently data prior to 1992 for both Northern and North West regions
   shown in this table in previous editions of RASER are not comparable with the 1993 data presented above.

12 Accidents on trunk 'A' roads: by carriageway type, junction, number of lanes, region[1] and severity: 1993

Number of accidents

	Dual carriageway					Single carriageway							Circular section of round-about[5]	All trunk A roads[6]
	Junction		Non-junction			Junction			Non-junction					
	Number of lanes[2]		Number of lanes[2]			Number of lanes[3]			Number of lanes[3]					
	2	3+	2	3+	All	2[4]	3	4+	2[4]	3	4+	All		
Northern[7]														
Fatal or serious	25	3	37	2	67	28	2	0	88	1	1	120	5	193
All severities	139	18	203	38	398	218	12	4	266	7	2	509	78	987
Yorkshire and Humberside														
Fatal or serious	42	3	64	1	110	83	7	3	102	6	2	203	11	324
All severities	165	9	238	12	424	343	26	27	320	16	5	737	124	1,290
East Midlands														
Fatal or serious	60	4	87	4	155	121	4	5	144	3	5	282	26	463
All severities	234	22	330	11	597	543	38	28	470	10	17	1,106	232	1,937
Eastern														
Fatal or serious	94	15	124	17	250	109	8	2	149	2	0	270	33	555
All severities	316	44	552	58	970	520	30	9	490	8	5	1,062	281	2,319
South East														
Fatal or serious	39	11	90	29	169	67	7	0	88	5	1	168	19	360
All severities	226	62	438	137	863	366	20	5	315	18	5	729	251	1,863
London														
Fatal or serious	88	126	63	107	384	116	8	55	38	3	8	228	26	643
All severities	526	728	376	498	2,128	937	60	373	293	23	83	1,769	275	4,230
of which:														
Inner London														
Fatal or serious	14	54	12	25	105	64	3	40	21	0	6	134	7	249
All severities	143	255	74	116	588	536	28	260	140	10	53	1,027	33	1,676
Outer London														
Fatal or serious	74	72	51	82	279	52	5	15	17	3	2	94	19	394
All severities	383	473	302	382	1,540	401	32	113	153	13	30	742	242	2,554
South West														
Fatal or serious	20	1	45	7	73	72	5	3	85	12	0	177	13	263
All severities	90	9	171	19	289	371	20	5	386	39	1	822	164	1,286
West Midlands														
Fatal or serious	39	5	42	4	90	94	13	3	101	2	1	214	26	330
All severities	215	17	231	14	477	409	27	5	341	8	2	792	244	1,515
North West[7]														
Fatal or serious	36	18	29	7	90	43	5	13	55	3	8	127	11	228
All severities	234	128	135	33	530	327	22	95	223	11	42	720	143	1,409
England														
Fatal or serious	443	186	581	178	1,388	733	59	84	850	37	26	1,789	170	3,359
All severities	2,145	1,037	2,674	820	6,676	4,034	255	551	3,104	140	162	8,246	1,792	16,836
Wales														
Fatal or serious	28	2	29	0	59	83	9	0	161	13	0	266	8	333
All severities	105	14	196	4	319	380	32	0	530	38	0	980	87	1,390
Scotland														
Fatal or serious	79	2	83	5	169	134	4	5	284	5	5	437	7	614
All severities	220	15	321	21	577	456	12	11	858	13	15	1,365	59	2,005
Great Britain														
Fatal or serious	550	190	693	183	1,616	950	72	89	1,295	55	31	2,492	185	4,306
All severities	2,470	1,066	3,191	845	7,572	4,870	299	562	4,492	191	177	10,591	1,938	20,231

1 Accident data in this breakdown are not available for Northern Ireland.
2 Number of lanes in each direction.
3 Number of lanes in both directions.
4 Includes one way streets.
5 These are classified as junction accidents.
6 Includes unknown carriageway type and single track roads.
7 From 1st April 1991 responsibilty for Cumbria transferred from the North West Regional Office to the Northern Regional Office. The change to the road accident database was deferred until 1992. Consequently data prior to 1992 for both Northern and North West regions shown in this table in previous editions of RASER are not comparable with the 1993 data presented above.

13 Accidents on principal 'A' roads: by carriageway type, junction, number of lanes, region[1] and severity: 1993

Number of accidents

	Dual carriageway					Single carriageway							Circular section of round-about[5]	All principal A roads[6]
	Junction		Non-junction			Junction			Non-junction					
	Number of lanes[2]		Number of lanes[2]			Number of lanes[3]			Number of lanes[3]					
	2	3+	2	3+	All	2[4]	3	4+	2[4]	3	4+	All		
Northern[7]														
Fatal or serious	45	7	44	7	103	206	13	17	229	9	11	485	30	624
All severities	259	34	197	22	512	1,245	71	83	911	25	54	2,389	328	3,270
Yorkshire and Humberside														
Fatal or serious	107	26	95	12	240	495	43	19	504	16	7	1,084	52	1,381
All severities	704	157	362	57	1,280	2,717	217	136	1,816	56	35	4,977	535	6,828
East Midlands														
Fatal or serious	52	14	45	4	115	411	16	42	459	10	22	960	47	1,125
All severities	297	69	217	18	601	2,236	98	246	1,684	31	85	4,380	390	5,395
Eastern														
Fatal or serious	97	11	86	8	202	566	30	12	581	23	2	1,214	82	1,503
All severities	556	59	423	31	1,069	3,177	188	78	2,173	93	20	5,729	994	7,843
South East														
Fatal or serious	143	16	122	13	294	730	40	36	661	18	13	1,498	101	1,923
All severities	831	129	617	53	1,630	4,450	226	228	2,770	67	72	7,813	1,178	10,811
London														
Fatal or serious	238	59	87	11	395	1,494	63	261	558	18	73	2,467	67	2,959
All severities	1,435	336	465	93	2,329	10,494	354	1,808	3,187	90	440	16,373	613	19,565
of which:														
Inner London														
Fatal or serious	142	38	46	8	234	718	37	176	242	9	57	1,239	22	1,522
All severities	832	212	233	64	1,341	5,332	191	1,245	1,425	53	334	8,580	233	10,306
Outer London														
Fatal or serious	96	21	41	3	161	776	26	85	316	9	16	1,228	45	1,437
All severities	603	124	232	29	988	5,162	163	563	1,762	37	106	7,793	380	9,259
South West														
Fatal or serious	57	10	53	7	127	440	24	5	497	15	2	983	59	1,181
All severities	324	65	242	30	661	2,472	114	33	1,994	49	19	4,681	582	6,003
West Midlands														
Fatal or serious	106	43	102	20	271	472	26	69	377	12	26	982	60	1,316
All severities	742	213	434	55	1,444	2,807	145	345	1,587	57	99	5,040	681	7,194
North West[7]														
Fatal or serious	130	80	77	37	324	668	44	133	402	10	42	1,299	31	1,666
All severities	1,314	632	489	175	2,610	5,238	289	868	1,973	38	186	8,592	455	11,909
England														
Fatal or serious	975	266	711	119	2,071	5,482	299	594	4,268	131	198	10,972	529	13,678
All severities	6,462	1,694	3,446	534	12,136	34,836	1,702	3,825	18,095	506	1,010	59,974	5,756	78,818
Wales														
Fatal or serious	29	7	16	3	55	181	19	10	270	9	3	492	22	571
All severities	208	48	122	15	393	1,127	98	66	1,099	33	17	2,440	253	3,121
Scotland														
Fatal or serious	77	20	92	13	202	362	10	48	637	5	36	1,098	21	1,344
All severities	394	98	368	64	924	1,750	65	271	2,152	19	158	4,415	240	5,657
Great Britain														
Fatal or serious	1,081	293	819	135	2,328	6,025	328	652	5,175	145	237	12,562	572	15,593
All severities	7,064	1,840	3,936	613	13,453	37,713	1,865	4,162	21,346	558	1,185	66,829	6,249	87,596

1 Accident data in this breakdown are not available for Northern Ireland.
2 Number of lanes in each direction.
3 Number of lanes in both directions.
4 Includes one way streets.
5 These are classified as junction accidents.
6 Includes unknown carriageway type and single track roads.
7 From 1st April 1991 responsibilty for Cumbria transferred from the North West Regional Office to the Northern Regional Office.
  The change to the road accident database was deferred until 1992. Consequently data prior to 1992 for both Northern and North West regions shown in
  this table in previous editions of RASER are not comparable with the 1993 data presented above.

33

14 Accidents: by road class, severity, region and county: 1981-85 average, 1992, 1993

Number

	Motorways			Trunk A roads			Principal A roads			All roads		
	Fatal	Fatal or serious	All severities	Fatal	Fatal or serious	All severities	Fatal	Fatal or serious	All severities	Fatal	Fatal or serious	All severities
Northern Region[1]												
1981-85	7	37	118	34	259	833	104	1,009	3,602	260	2,930	10,613
1992	8	34	178	47	245	1,062	67	669	3,368	202	2,134	10,510
1993	9	36	186	43	193	987	74	624	3,270	211	1,876	9,936
Cleveland[2]												
1981-85	0	0	0	4	19	97	18	174	770	42	423	2,137
1992	0	0	0	1	13	97	12	119	710	24	338	1,996
1993	0	0	0	5	19	128	9	102	673	27	322	1,931
Cumbria[1]												
1981-85	5	22	62	13	127	355	16	195	605	55	675	2,043
1992	5	22	83	21	107	367	14	128	516	59	452	1,780
1993	2	18	70	23	101	378	14	118	550	53	386	1,818
Durham												
1981-85	2	10	35	7	40	110	24	195	585	55	577	1,801
1992	1	6	60	5	39	179	16	106	586	40	360	2,041
1993	6	12	74	4	12	135	11	86	520	36	273	1,882
Northumberland[2]												
1981-85	0	0	0	7	45	163	11	87	280	35	313	1,043
1992	0	0	0	13	56	201	12	68	312	31	224	1,008
1993	0	0	0	9	42	173	11	72	357	32	226	1,024
Tyne and Wear												
1981-85	0	5	21	2	29	107	36	357	1,361	73	942	3,588
1992	2	6	35	7	30	218	13	248	1,244	48	760	3,685
1993	1	6	42	2	19	173	29	246	1,170	63	669	3,281
Yorkshire and Humberside Region												
1981-85	14	78	306	65	541	1,498	196	2,053	6,932	463	5,714	20,018
1992	17	98	514	43	419	1,478	158	1,514	6,814	373	4,231	19,714
1993	17	77	518	43	324	1,290	156	1,381	6,828	351	3,810	19,276
Humberside												
1981-85	2	10	33	8	72	243	28	308	1,201	73	996	3,894
1992	5	15	58	5	59	226	30	253	1,074	78	850	3,872
1993	1	12	55	8	42	192	21	247	1,026	61	817	3,582
North Yorkshire												
1981-85	0	3	8	24	239	467	29	474	1,048	82	1,423	3,128
1992	1	5	8	16	194	493	24	351	1,043	71	1,013	3,048
1993	1	1	4	21	175	481	30	349	1,076	82	988	3,078
South Yorkshire												
1981-85	4	26	110	10	75	250	42	420	1,654	103	1,123	4,631
1992	5	31	183	10	53	246	39	279	1,557	86	721	4,407
1993	5	20	190	6	27	159	40	244	1,645	79	604	4,558
West Yorkshire												
1981-85	7	39	155	23	155	538	96	851	3,030	205	2,172	8,365
1992	6	47	265	12	113	513	65	631	3,140	138	1,647	8,387
1993	10	44	269	8	80	458	65	541	3,081	129	1,401	8,058
East Midlands Region												
1981-85	15	129	390	97	792	2,350	158	1,770	5,721	443	5,334	17,379
1992	16	73	361	88	508	2,061	119	1,164	5,493	346	3,388	16,051
1993	11	87	450	76	463	1,937	119	1,125	5,395	319	3,289	15,850
Derbyshire												
1981-85	2	18	69	20	159	545	34	339	1,130	97	1,057	3,743
1992	5	18	91	20	129	563	17	155	1,090	69	545	3,551
1993	2	14	112	21	100	507	26	146	1,077	69	477	3,504
Leicestershire												
1981-85	6	24	93	16	115	360	32	330	1,198	93	1,042	3,702
1992	8	22	124	15	68	275	27	189	1,216	81	593	3,453
1993	4	24	143	13	55	294	28	181	1,199	76	545	3,452

1 From 1st April 1991 responsibilty for Cumbria transferred from the North West Regional Office to the Northern Regional Office.
   The change to the road accident database was deferred until 1992. However, for this table, data prior to 1992 have been changed to take account of the new boundaries.
2 This county contains no motorways.

34

14 Accidents: by road class, severity, region and county: 1981-85 average, 1992, 1993 (cont.)

	Motorways			Trunk A roads			Principal A roads			All roads		
	Fatal	Fatal or serious	All severities	Fatal	Fatal or serious	All severities	Fatal	Fatal or serious	All severities	Fatal	Fatal or serious	All severities
Lincolnshire[1]												
1981-85	0	0	0	20	160	454	29	294	932	76	852	2,683
1992	0	0	0	18	81	327	30	260	913	62	624	2,440
1993	0	0	0	14	84	279	27	255	923	65	641	2,439
Northamptonshire												
1981-85	6	75	190	18	182	434	22	381	1,011	69	1,025	2,673
1992	2	22	101	16	90	306	26	225	854	58	587	2,227
1993	4	38	138	8	77	290	15	226	848	41	599	2,211
Nottinghamshire												
1981-85	1	11	38	22	175	557	41	426	1,450	108	1,359	4,577
1992	1	11	45	19	140	590	19	335	1,420	76	1,039	4,380
1993	1	11	57	20	147	567	23	317	1,348	68	1,027	4,244
Eastern Region												
1981-85	20	153	560	104	876	2,591	199	2,488	8,215	543	7,727	25,186
1992	22	165	967	66	563	2,411	175	1,541	7,629	434	5,054	24,208
1993	24	177	1,059	88	555	2,319	158	1,503	7,843	427	4,697	24,016
Bedfordshire												
1981-85	4	29	109	10	94	345	17	160	622	50	600	2,444
1992	5	22	113	8	52	297	17	96	544	45	375	2,111
1993	1	13	92	12	58	281	13	92	582	44	341	2,036
Buckinghamshire												
1981-85	5	38	120	3	36	110	27	318	1,001	63	843	2,617
1992	8	26	201	3	13	110	26	139	911	59	402	2,744
1993	3	30	235	3	16	111	24	116	861	51	345	2,624
Cambridgeshire												
1981-85	1	5	19	23	158	462	25	303	1,009	75	908	2,979
1992	1	2	22	13	127	522	30	262	1,149	63	797	3,389
1993	1	7	22	14	117	444	24	242	1,089	60	716	3,279
Essex												
1981-85	3	29	109	11	97	321	53	675	2,398	125	2,032	6,976
1992	2	39	225	13	82	403	30	351	2,037	83	1,132	6,322
1993	7	49	237	14	95	469	38	356	2,090	88	1,147	6,364
Hertfordshire												
1981-85	7	53	203	16	121	404	30	393	1,469	84	1,177	4,316
1992	6	76	406	7	73	305	22	251	1,162	57	898	3,991
1993	12	78	473	8	74	308	19	279	1,352	56	880	4,219
Norfolk[1]												
1981-85	0	0	0	21	190	461	27	360	910	82	1,207	3,110
1992	0	0	0	14	123	415	36	253	1,084	95	884	3,387
1993	0	0	0	21	116	391	29	265	1,150	84	792	3,301
Suffolk[1]												
1981-85	0	0	0	20	179	488	19	280	805	64	960	2,744
1992	0	0	0	8	93	359	14	189	742	32	566	2,264
1993	0	0	0	16	79	315	11	153	719	44	476	2,193
South East Region												
1981-85	29	205	652	109	800	2,453	282	3,500	12,091	677	9,327	32,192
1992	40	223	1,281	55	426	2,053	184	2,062	11,017	463	5,415	29,152
1993	20	234	1,373	59	360	1,863	183	1,923	10,811	427	5,010	28,371
Berkshire												
1981-85	10	69	215	7	61	195	24	321	1,167	71	942	3,263
1992	7	39	241	1	10	95	10	135	1,081	41	359	2,816
1993	2	31	224	1	11	113	15	141	1,057	30	336	2,770
East Sussex[1]												
1981-85	0	0	0	10	78	232	31	347	1,163	66	838	2,997
1992	0	0	0	5	44	198	21	196	1,082	49	482	2,742
1993	0	0	0	7	53	200	19	204	1,077	51	514	2,701

1 This county contains no motorways.

Number

	Motorways			Trunk A roads			Principal A roads			All roads		
	Fatal	Fatal or serious	All severities	Fatal	Fatal or serious	All severities	Fatal	Fatal or serious	All severities	Fatal	Fatal or serious	All severities
Hampshire												
1981-85	4	36	109	21	160	437	50	792	2,416	140	2,320	7,227
1992	3	45	208	5	64	273	37	482	2,184	96	1,385	6,643
1993	2	60	276	12	64	261	40	425	2,283	103	1,248	6,692
Isle of Wight[1]												
1981-85	0	0	0	0	0	0	4	70	214	8	155	495
1992	0	0	0	0	0	0	3	54	180	5	115	421
1993	0	0	0	0	0	0	2	35	160	6	89	392
Kent												
1981-85	7	49	162	21	175	539	63	779	2,543	142	2,053	6,819
1992	12	49	248	21	150	606	49	473	2,341	114	1,331	6,185
1993	4	42	273	15	98	517	33	488	2,296	84	1,198	5,910
Oxfordshire												
1981-85	1	6	12	24	164	521	26	279	801	71	871	2,531
1992	6	20	91	11	65	359	23	158	821	53	408	2,303
1993	6	22	118	8	43	285	22	131	816	47	343	2,222
Surrey												
1981-85	7	43	144	10	62	224	52	613	2,618	109	1,391	5,870
1992	11	67	471	7	44	251	24	355	2,249	64	858	5,297
1993	5	77	467	4	39	241	31	334	2,134	56	828	5,136
West Sussex												
1981-85	0	2	9	16	102	306	31	299	1,170	70	757	2,990
1992	1	3	22	5	49	271	17	209	1,079	41	477	2,745
1993	1	2	15	12	52	246	21	165	988	50	454	2,548
London												
1981-85	6	35	266	56	413	2,489	301	4,269	25,584	521	7,588	45,274
1992	3	61	482	62	745	4,406	135	3,220	19,175	308	6,575	38,748
1993	3	61	435	45	643	4,230	141	2,959	19,565	277	5,842	38,533
Inner London												
1981-85[2]	..	..	..	..	..	..	..	..	..	212	3,383	20,946
1992	1	9	60	17	287	1,735	58	1,606	10,087	112	2,949	18,100
1993	0	3	39	13	249	1,676	67	1,522	10,306	116	2,659	18,000
Outer London												
1981-85[2]	..	..	..	..	..	..	..	..	..	309	4,204	24,327
1992	2	52	422	45	458	2,671	77	1,614	9,088	196	3,626	20,648
1993	3	58	396	32	394	2,554	74	1,437	9,259	161	3,183	20,533
South West Region												
1981-85	17	127	344	62	585	1,586	197	2,475	7,390	440	6,697	19,847
1992	13	77	370	55	276	1,303	140	1,275	5,824	335	3,425	16,380
1993	10	68	409	41	263	1,286	119	1,181	6,003	273	3,290	17,014
Avon												
1981-85	8	50	124	3	29	61	41	450	1,415	86	1,149	3,596
1992	5	23	150	3	16	49	27	170	827	65	480	2,629
1993	6	25	183	2	13	51	19	170	945	48	485	2,857
Cornwall[1]												
1981-85	0	0	0	10	92	249	14	236	667	39	696	1,984
1992	0	0	0	11	50	250	15	127	585	37	368	1,770
1993	0	0	0	4	37	225	16	136	678	31	357	1,966
Devon												
1981-85	2	10	27	13	131	345	35	570	1,563	82	1,568	4,354
1992	2	14	51	12	61	298	17	291	1,139	55	863	3,690
1993	0	12	46	10	66	292	16	227	1,156	44	804	3,957
Dorset[1]												
1981-85	0	0	0	4	45	148	23	311	1,112	48	803	2,779
1992	0	0	0	6	23	148	24	182	1,034	47	428	2,427
1993	0	0	0	6	32	147	21	158	999	47	422	2,450

1 This county contains no motorways.
2 Trunk road data are not available for these years.

14 Accidents: by road class, severity, region and county: 1981-85 average, 1992, 1993 (cont.)

	Motorways			Trunk A roads			Principal A roads			All roads		
	Fatal	Fatal or serious	All severities	Fatal	Fatal or serious	All severities	Fatal	Fatal or serious	All severities	Fatal	Fatal or serious	All severities
Gloucestershire												
1981-85	1	21	54	13	145	369	24	282	705	59	967	2,479
1992	2	7	52	9	50	269	11	141	692	43	386	2,051
1993	0	5	54	8	39	255	15	131	679	35	376	2,039
Somerset												
1981-85	3	17	43	6	48	117	29	295	789	57	666	1,783
1992	1	9	46	4	14	60	24	167	710	40	372	1,646
1993	1	9	47	3	16	70	18	156	681	30	335	1,530
Wiltshire												
1981-85	4	28	96	12	94	297	32	331	1,138	68	847	2,871
1992	3	24	71	10	62	229	22	197	837	48	528	2,167
1993	3	17	79	8	60	246	14	203	865	38	511	2,215
West Midlands Region												
1981-85	19	138	476	81	639	1,827	190	2,263	7,415	484	6,527	21,030
1992	19	147	719	59	377	1,601	150	1,462	7,196	357	4,137	20,130
1993	21	160	788	47	330	1,515	129	1,316	7,194	307	3,769	19,783
Hereford and Worcester												
1981-85	4	29	104	10	83	245	31	329	1,060	71	859	2,762
1992	3	24	116	10	63	321	28	197	899	53	509	2,534
1993	3	17	101	10	55	249	26	181	918	55	432	2,446
Shropshire												
1981-85	0	2	4	14	147	363	17	170	473	51	653	1,611
1992	1	1	9	12	85	242	18	132	465	49	406	1,546
1993	1	7	16	16	73	213	10	102	441	41	370	1,521
Staffordshire												
1981-85	8	36	146	25	163	602	36	405	1,577	105	1,209	4,813
1992	1	19	208	17	104	582	29	216	1,611	72	632	4,679
1993	4	19	260	9	82	558	32	199	1,680	63	569	4,686
Warwickshire												
1981-85	4	29	68	19	148	336	23	220	553	77	850	2,078
1992	7	51	171	14	76	236	13	171	616	48	665	2,246
1993	3	67	197	7	76	249	9	137	616	28	585	2,250
West Midlands												
1981-85	4	41	154	12	98	280	84	1,140	3,752	180	2,956	9,767
1992	7	52	215	6	49	220	62	746	3,605	135	1,925	9,125
1993	10	50	214	5	44	246	52	697	3,539	120	1,813	8,880
North West Region[1]												
1981-85	29	158	749	48	314	1,252	232	2,208	10,622	503	5,504	26,599
1992	37	158	1,235	32	206	1,439	190	1,729	11,906	408	4,250	29,648
1993	25	147	1,209	22	228	1,409	180	1,666	11,909	352	4,168	29,363
Cheshire												
1981-85	8	44	198	17	92	400	32	277	1,436	83	778	3,913
1992	9	45	343	10	49	388	29	212	1,459	73	540	3,951
1993	8	32	353	6	69	402	41	204	1,537	75	520	4,137
Greater Manchester												
1981-85	10	59	337	6	50	214	90	971	4,966	178	2,149	11,127
1992	16	58	543	2	24	233	82	720	5,462	153	1,613	12,510
1993	9	48	491	3	23	219	66	663	5,424	132	1,497	12,196
Lancashire												
1981-85	8	40	147	17	113	377	60	554	2,161	135	1,478	5,803
1992	7	39	207	15	95	447	46	412	2,212	109	1,133	6,058
1993	6	53	222	7	90	396	41	460	2,168	81	1,281	5,822
Merseyside												
1981-85	3	14	67	7	59	260	50	406	2,059	107	1,099	5,756
1992	5	16	142	5	38	371	33	385	2,773	73	964	7,129
1993	2	14	143	6	46	392	32	339	2,780	64	870	7,208

1 From 1st April 1991 responsibilty for Cumbria transferred from the North West Regional Office to the Northern Regional Office.
The change to the road accident database was deferred until 1992. However, for this table, data prior to 1992 have been changed to take account of the new boundaries.

14 Accidents: by road class, severity, region and county: 1981-85 average, 1992, 1993 (cont.)

	Motorways			Trunk A roads			Principal A roads			All roads		
	Fatal	Fatal or serious	All severities	Fatal	Fatal or serious	All severities	Fatal	Fatal or serious	All severities	Fatal	Fatal or serious	All severities
England												
1981-85	156	1,059	3,860	654	5,220	16,880	1,859	22,035	87,572	4,333	57,347	218,137
1992	175	1,036	6,107	507	3,765	17,814	1,318	14,636	78,422	3,226	38,609	204,541
1993	140	1,047	6,427	464	3,359	16,836	1,259	13,678	78,818	2,944	35,751	202,142
Wales												
1981-85	5	38	124	62	620	1,746	86	984	3,427	233	3,082	10,583
1992	3	28	162	54	385	1,475	73	676	3,308	206	2,033	10,467
1993	2	17	153	43	333	1,390	61	571	3,121	167	1,747	10,049
Scotland												
1981-85	16	110	265	138	1,010	2,433	228	2,751	7,438	581	7,412	20,471
1992	13	85	361	119	718	2,142	145	1,597	6,073	423	4,696	18,017
1993	17	74	283	93	614	2,005	131	1,344	5,657	359	4,003	16,674
Great Britain												
1981-85	177	1,207	4,249	854	6,850	21,058	2,173	25,769	98,436	5,147	67,842	249,192
1992	191	1,149	6,630	680	4,868	21,431	1,536	16,909	87,803	3,855	45,338	233,025
1993	159	1,138	6,863	600	4,306	20,231	1,451	15,593	87,596	3,470	41,501	228,865

15 Accidents and casualties by severity: vehicles involved by vehicle type: road length: all by selected individual motorways[1]: 1993

	Accidents			Casualties			Vehicles involved				Kilo-metres open at December 1993[3]
	Fatal	Serious	All severities	Fatal	Serious	All severities	Two-wheel motor vehicles	Cars and LGV	HGV	All vehicles[2]	
England											
M1, M10	23	134	956	26	180	1,623	40	1,775	343	2,189	307
M45	0	1	2	0	2	4	0	3	0	3	13
M2	1	10	70	10	19	170	3	102	31	141	43
M3	1	52	201	2	70	337	18	370	47	439	88
M4	9	87	610	12	110	936	34	1,248	126	1,432	188
M5	7	52	340	8	68	536	13	560	98	683	263
M6	20	139	966	21	198	1,572	31	1,847	414	2,315	391
M11	6	25	145	6	35	225	8	222	59	296	85
M18	2	6	43	2	6	60	2	63	11	76	45
M20	3	16	114	3	21	156	8	172	40	224	82
M23	2	12	82	3	15	151	0	173	10	193	27
M25	9	111	833	9	143	1,332	49	1,678	251	2,001	190
M26	0	1	6	0	2	14	0	16	0	16	17
M27, M271, M275	2	26	157	2	36	225	17	285	23	328	52
M40	7	44	261	19	68	420	8	428	67	505	146
M42	2	27	115	2	39	195	4	212	42	259	68
M50	2	3	21	6	9	36	0	22	10	32	34
M53	2	6	67	2	7	93	4	112	3	121	33
M54	1	7	29	2	9	41	2	39	3	44	36
M55	1	4	18	1	6	34	1	33	2	36	19
M56	2	7	125	2	7	178	2	241	40	289	58
M57	0	3	26	0	3	38	0	42	5	50	17
M58	0	1	18	0	1	30	2	24	2	28	19
M61	0	11	69	0	13	111	1	130	14	145	39
M62	14	48	403	15	61	648	15	704	164	897	167
M63	1	2	83	1	2	117	2	149	23	174	25
M65	1	2	24	1	4	35	0	39	2	41	13
M66	1	5	44	1	6	69	0	75	11	86	19
M69	1	6	24	1	8	37	0	32	3	35	27
M180 & M181	1	7	29	1	10	51	0	18	7	25	45
Other motorways	2	5	107	4	5	150	8	219	20	248	42
Motorways	123	860	5,988	162	1,163	9,624	272	11,033	1,871	13,351	2,598
A(M) roads	17	47	439	19	70	702	33	824	80	953	158
Total (inc A(M) roads)	140	907	6,427	181	1,233	10,326	305	11,857	1,951	14,304	2,756
Wales											
Motorways	2	14	149	2	17	229	7	275	32	314	120
A(M) roads	0	1	4	0	1	4	0	6	0	6	4
Total (inc A(M) roads)	2	15	153	2	18	233	7	281	32	320	124
Scotland											
Motorways	17	56	282	18	86	486	11	413	62	498	279[4]
A(M) roads	0	1	1	0	1	1	0	1	1	2	6[4]
Total (inc A(M) roads)	17	57	283	18	87	487	11	414	63	500	286[5]
Great Britain											
Motorways	142	930	6,419	182	1,266	10,339	290	11,721	1,965	14,163	2,718
A(M) roads	17	49	444	19	72	707	33	831	81	961	162
Total (inc A(M) roads)	159	979	6,863	201	1,338	11,046	323	12,552	2,046	15,124	2,880

1 Motorway accident data are not available in this breakdown for Northern Ireland.
2 Includes pedal cycles, buses and coaches and other vehicles.
3 Excluding slip roads. Data for England from DOT Highways Computing Division. Data for Wales from Welsh Office and Scotland from Scottish Office.
4 As at December 1992.
5 As at 1 April 1994.

16 Distribution of accidents by road class and region [1] : 1992, 1993

percentage (row sums = 100)

	Motorways		Trunk roads		Principal roads		Other roads	
	1992	1993	1992	1993	1992	1993	1992	1993
Northern [2]	1.7	1.9	10.1	9.9	32.0	32.9	56.2	55.3
Yorkshire and Humberside	2.6	2.7	7.5	6.7	34.6	35.4	55.3	55.2
East Midlands	2.2	2.8	12.8	12.2	34.2	34.0	50.7	50.9
Eastern	4.0	4.4	10.0	9.7	31.5	32.7	54.5	53.3
South Eastern	4.4	4.8	7.0	6.6	37.8	38.1	50.8	50.5
London	1.2	1.1	11.4	11.0	49.5	50.8	37.9	37.1
South West	2.3	2.4	8.0	7.6	35.5	35.3	54.2	54.8
West Midlands	3.6	4.0	8.0	7.7	35.7	36.4	52.7	52.0
North West [2]	4.2	4.1	4.9	4.8	40.2	40.6	50.8	50.5
England	3.0	3.2	8.7	8.3	38.3	39.0	50.0	49.5
Wales	1.5	1.5	14.1	13.8	31.6	31.1	52.8	53.6
Scotland	2.0	1.7	11.9	12.0	33.7	33.9	52.4	52.4
Great Britain	2.8	3.0	9.2	8.8	37.7	38.3	50.3	49.9

1   Accident data in this breakdown are not available for Northern Ireland.
2   From 1st April 1991 responsibilty for Cumbria transferred from the North West Regional Office to the Northern Regional Office.
    The change to the road accident database was deferred until 1992. Consequently, the data prior to 1992 for both the Northern and North West regions
    shown in this table in previous editions of RASER are not comparable with the 1993 data presented above.

17 Motor vehicles, population, area and road length (motorways and built-up and non built-up roads: by trunk and principal): by region: 1993

Thousands/ number

	Motor vehicles currently licensed [1] (thousands)	Population [2] mid year (home) (thousands)	Area in hectares (thousands)	Road length (kilometres)				
				Motorways [3]	Built-up [4]		Non built-up [4]	
					Trunk	Principal	Trunk	Principal
Northern [5]	1,108	3,099	1,540	152	55	610	749	1,436
Yorkshire and Humberside	2,027	5,002	1,542	290	131	1,165	672	1,407
East Midlands	1,738	4,062	1,563	185	153	774	1,089	1,959
Eastern	2,946	5,821	2,100	316	103	1,108	1,209	2,352
South East	3,458	7,067	1,722	567	76	1,616	798	2,426
London	2,674	6,905	158	60	207	1,353	134	44
South West	2,383	4,746	2,385	302	54	1,115	994	2,872
West Midlands	2,463	5,277	1,301	380	102	1,145	750	1,603
North West [5]	2,554	6,400	733	486	99	1,682	407	974
England	21,352	48,378	13,044	2,737	981	10,568	6,801	15,074
Wales	1,174	2,899	2,077	124	211	850	1,368	1,804
Scotland	1,874	5,111	7,717	286	216	1,271	2,653	6,636
Great Britain	24,826	56,388	22,838	3,147	1,408	12,689	10,822	23,514
Northern Ireland	586	1,610	1,412	112	284	216	869	856
United Kingdom	25,412	57,998	24,250	3,259	1,692	12,905	11,691	24,370

1   Includes all vehicles licensed to use public roads. From 1992, estimates of licensed stock are taken from the Department of Transport's Statistics Directorate
    Information Database.
2   Final 1992 population estimates.
3   Excluding slip roads. Data for England from DOT Highways Computing Division. Total for England includes figures for non-trunk motorways
    not included in regional totals. Data for Wales from Welsh Office and Scotland from Scottish Office.
4   As at April 1993. Road length figures taken from DOT Transport Statistics Report "Road Lengths in Great Britain 1993".
5   From 1st April 1991 responsibilty for Cumbria transferred from the North West Regional Office to the Northern Regional Office.
    Consequently, the data prior to 1992 for both the Northern and North West regions shown in this table in previous editions of RASER are not comparable
    with the 1993 data presented above.

18 Motor traffic distribution between regions [1] : by motorway and built-up and non built-up trunk and principal roads: 1991-1993 average

percentage [2]

	Motorways	Built-up 'A'		Non built-up 'A'		All major roads
		Trunk	Principal	Trunk	Principal	
Northern [3]	2	2	4	6	6	4
Yorkshire & Humberside	8	7	9	8	7	8
East Midlands	6	10	5	10	9	8
Eastern	14	7	8	17	16	13
South East	21	7	13	14	18	16
London	2	33	15	5	0	7
South West	9	4	8	9	14	10
West Midlands	13	9	10	7	8	9
North West [3]	16	7	15	5	7	11
England	92	85	88	81	84	86
Wales	3	8	4	7	5	5
Scotland	5	7	7	12	10	9
Great Britain	100	100	100	100	100	100

1 Traffic data are not available for Northern Ireland.
2 Figures have been rounded to the nearest whole number.
3 From 1st April 1991 responsibilty for Cumbria transferred from the North West Regional Office to the Northern Regional Office. The change to the road accident database was deferred until 1992.

19 Motor traffic distribution between motorways, built-up and non built-up trunk and principal roads: by region [1] : 1991-1993 average

percentage [2]

	Motorways	Built-up 'A'		Non built-up 'A'		All major roads
		Trunk	Principal	Trunk	Principal	
Northern [3]	13	2	24	31	31	100
Yorkshire & Humberside	24	3	31	22	20	100
East Midlands	19	5	19	31	26	100
Eastern	26	2	17	29	26	100
South East	31	2	22	20	25	100
London	7	17	58	17	2	100
South West	21	2	23	22	33	100
West Midlands	33	3	29	16	18	100
North West [3]	35	2	37	11	14	100
England	25	4	27	22	22	100
Wales	14	6	23	33	25	100
Scotland	15	3	23	32	27	100
Great Britain	24	4	27	23	23	100

1 Traffic data are not available for Northern Ireland.
2 Figures have been rounded to the nearest whole number.
3 From 1st April 1991 responsibilty for Cumbria transferred from the North West Regional Office to the Northern Regional Office. The change to the road accident database was deferred until 1992.

41

Definitions

Accident: One involving personal injury occurring on the public highway (including footways) in which a road vehicle is involved and which becomes known to the police within 30 days of its occurrence. The vehicle need not be moving and it need not be in collision with anything. One accident may give rise to several *casualties*. Damage-only accidents are not included in this publication.

'A' Roads: All purpose *trunk* roads and *principal* local authority roads.

Adults: Persons aged 16 years and over.

Built-up Roads: Roads with speed limits (ignoring temporary limits) of 40 mph or less. The pre-1982 definition of 'built-up areas' referred to the same roads but the general nature of the area was never relevant. 'Non built-up roads' refer to those with speed limits of over 40 mph. *Motorways* are included with non built-up roads unless otherwise stated. In tables where data for *motorways* are shown separately, the totals for built-up and non built-up roads exclude *motorway accidents*. In comparing such tables with those involving a built-up/non built-up split only, negligible error will be made by assuming that *motorway accidents* were all on non built-up roads.

Cars: Includes taxis, estate cars, invalid tricycles, three and four-wheeled cars, minibuses and motor caravans.

Casualty: A person *killed* or injured in an *accident*. Casualties are classified as either *killed, seriously injured* or *slightly injured*.

Children: Persons under 16 years of age.

Fatal Accident: One in which at least one person is *killed* (but excluding confirmed suicides).

Heavy goods vehicles (HGV): Those over 1.524 tonnes unladen weight. Includes vehicles with six or more tyres and some four-wheel vehicles with extra large bodies and larger rear tyres. Includes a tractor unit travelling without its usual trailer. From 1 January 1994 the weight definition changed to those vehicles over 3.5 tonnes maximum permissible gross vehicle weight (gvw) and these vehicles will be called 'goods vehicles'.

Light goods vehicles (LGV): Vehicles not over 1.524 tonnes unladen weight. Light vans mainly include vehicles of the van type constructed on a car chassis. From 1 January 1994 the weight definition changed to those vehicles not over 3.5 tonnes maximum permissible gross vehicle weight and these vehicles will continue to be called 'light goods vehicles'.

Killed: Human *casualties* who sustained injuries resulting in death within 30 days of the *accident*.

KSI: *Killed* or *seriously injured*.

Licensed Vehicles: The stock of vehicles currently licensed on 31 December, when the annual census is taken at the Driver and Vehicle Licensing Agency (DVLA).

London: Where possible, data for London have been split into Inner and Outer London. Inner London comprises the City of London and the boroughs of Westminster, Camden, Islington, Hackney, Tower Hamlets, Lewisham, Southwark, Lambeth, Wandsworth, Hammersmith, Kensington and Chelsea, Newham and Haringey. Outer London is all other London boroughs, and includes Heathrow Airport. This definition conforms to that used by the Office of Population Censuses and Surveys (OPCS). See also *Regions*.

Major Roads: These are *motorways*, A(M) and *A class* roads (both *trunk* and *principal*).

Motorcyclist: Riders and passengers of two-wheeled motor vehicles.

Motorways: Motorways and A(M) roads except where otherwise noted. The motorway lengths given in Tables 15 and 17 are main line lengths and exclude associated slip roads.

Motorway Accident: *Accidents* on *motorways* include those on associated slip roads and those at junctions between *motorways* and other roads where the *accident* cannot be clearly allocated to the other road.

Other Roads: These are 'B' and 'C' class roads and unclassified roads, including 'road class not reported'.

Pedal cycle: Includes tandems, tricycles and toy cycles ridden on the carriageway. Also includes battery-assisted cycles and tricycles with a maximum speed of 15 mph.

Pedal cyclist: Riders of *pedal cycles* including any passengers.

Pedestrians: Also includes persons riding toy cycles on the footway, persons pushing bicycles or pushing or pulling other vehicles or operating pedestrian-controlled vehicles, those leading or herding animals, occupants of prams or wheelchairs, and persons who alight safely from vehicles and are subsequently injured.

Population: The population data used in calculating rates are the final mid-1992 estimates based on 1991 Census results. Mid-year estimates for 1993 were not available at the time of going to publication. The estimates include residents who are temporarily outside the country, and exclude both foreign visitors and members of HM armed forces who are stationed abroad.

Principal Roads: Roads for which County Councils (Regional and Island Authorities in Scotland) are the Highway Authority. The classified *principal roads* (which include local authority *motorways*) are those of regional and urban strategic importance.

Regions: In tables where data are disaggregated by region, Department of Transport (DOT) regions are used, as illustrated by the map on page 2. Greater London is not strictly a region and special arrangements apply, in that the responsibility falls to the London Regional Office (LRO) in DOT headquarters. The South East and Eastern regions do not include any of the Greater London area.

Serious Accident: One in which at least one person is *seriously injured* but no person (other than a confirmed suicide) is killed.

Serious Injury: An injury for which a person is detained in hospital as an 'in-patient', or any of the following injuries whether or not the *casualty* was detained in hospital: fractures, concussion, internal injuries, crushings, severe cuts and lacerations, severe general shock requiring medical treatment, injuries causing death 30 or more days after the *accident*. An injured *casualty* is coded as seriously or *slightly injured* by the police on the basis of information available within a short time of the *accident*. This generally will not include the result of a medical examination, but may include the fact of being detained in hospital, the reasons for which may vary from area to area.

Severity: Of an *accident*, the severity of the most severely injured *casualty* (either fatal, serious or slight); of a casualty, killed, seriously injured or slightly injured.

Slight Accident: One in which at least one person is *slightly injured*, but no person is *killed* or *seriously injured*.

Slight Injury: An injury of a minor character such as a sprain, bruise or cut which are not judged to be severe, or slight shock requiring roadside attention only.

Two-wheel motor vehicles: Mopeds, motor scooters and motor cycles (including motor cycle combinations.

Trunk Roads: Roads comprising the national network of through routes for which the Secretary of State for Transport in England and the Secretaries of State for Scotland and Wales are the highway authorities. The network contains both *motorways*, which legally are special roads reserved for certain classes of traffic, and all-purpose roads which are open to all classes of traffic.

Accident Record   Attendant Circumstances

1.1 Record Type   `1` 2
1 New accident record
5 Amended accident record

1.2 Police Force   3 4

1.3 Accident Ref No   5 6 7 8 9 10 11

1.4 Severity of Accident   12
1 Fatal 2 Serious 3 Slight

1.5 Number of Vehicles   13 14 15

1.6 Number of Casualty Records   16 17 18

1.7 Date
Day 19 20   Month 21 22   Year 23 24

1.8 Day of Week   25
1 Sunday   2 Monday
3 Tuesday   4 Wednesday
5 Thursday   6 Friday
7 Saturday

1.9 Time
Hrs 26 27   Mins 28 29
24 hour

1.10 Local Authority   30 31 32

1.11 Location
10 digit reference No
Easting 33 34 35 36 37
Northing 38 39 40 41 42

1.12 1st Road Class   43
1 Motorway
2 A (M)
3 A
4 B
5 C
6 Unclassified
7 } Local
8 } Authority
9 } Use Only

1.13 1st Road Number   44 45 46 47

1.14 Carriageway Type or Markings   48
1 Roundabout (on circular highway)
2 One way street
3 Dual carriageway - 2 lanes
4 Dual carriageway - 3 or more lanes
5 Single carriageway - single track road
6 Single carriageway - 2 lanes (one each direction)
7 Single carriageway - 3 lanes (two way capacity)
8 Single carriageway - 4 or more lanes (two way capacity)
9 Unknown

1.15 Speed Limit   49 `0` 50 51
mph

1.16 Junction Detail   52 `0` 53
0 Not at or within 20 metres of junction
1 Roundabout
2 Mini-roundabout
3 'T' or staggered junction
4 'Y' junction
5 Slip road
6 Crossroads
7 Multiple junction
8 Using private drive or entrance
9 Other junction

Junction Accidents Only

1.17 Junction Control   54
1 Authorised person
2 Automatic traffic signal
3 Stop sign
4 Give way sign or markings
5 Uncontrolled

1.18 2nd Road Class   55
1 Motorway
2 A (M)
3 A
4 B
5 C
6 Unclassified
7 } Local
8 } Authority
9 } Use Only

1.19 2nd Road Number   56 57 58 59

1.20 Pedestrian Crossing Facilities   60 `0` 61
0 No crossing facilities within 50 metres
1 Zebra
2 Zebra crossing controlled by school crossing patrol
3 Zebra crossing controlled by other authorised person
4 Pelican
5 Other light controlled crossing
6 Other sites controlled by school crossing patrol
7 Other sites controlled by other authorised person
8 Central refuge - no other controls
9 Footbridge or subway

1.21 Light Conditions   62
DAYLIGHT
1 Street lights 7 metres or more high
2 Street lights under 7 metres high
3 No street lighting
4 Daylight street lighting unknown
DARKNESS
5 Street lights 7 metres or more high (lit)
6 Street lights under 7 metres high (lit)
7 No street lighting
8 Street lights unlit
9 Darkness street lighting unknown

1.22 Weather   63
1 Fine (without high winds)
2 Raining (without high winds)
3 Snowing (without high winds)
4 Fine with high winds
5 Raining with high winds
6 Snowing with high winds
7 Fog (or mist if hazard)
8 Other
9 Unknown

1.23 Road Surface Condition   64
1 Dry
2 Wet/Damp
3 Snow
4 Frost/Ice
5 Flood (surface water over 3cms (1 inch) deep)

1.24 Special Conditions at Site   65
0 None
1 Automatic Traffic Signal-out
2 Automatic Traffic Signal partially defective
3 Permanent road signing defective or obscured
4 Road works present
5 Road surface defective

1.25 Carriageway Hazards   66
0 None
1 Dislodged vehicle load in carriageway
2 Other object in carriageway
3 Involvement with previous accident
4 Dog in carriageway
5 Other animal in carriageway

1.26 Overtaking Manoeuvre Patterns   67
No longer required by the Department of Transport

1.27 DTp Special Projects   68 69 70 71

Vehicle Record

2.1 Record Type
1 New vehicle record
5 Amended vehicle record

`1` `2` : `2`

2.2 Police Force

`3` `4`

2.3 Accident Ref No

`5` `6` `7` `8` `9` `10` `11`

2.4 Vehicle Ref No

`12` `13` `14`

2.5 Type of Vehicle

`15` `16`

01 Pedal cycle
02 Moped
03 Motor scooter
04 Motor cycle
05 Combination
06 Invalid Tricycle
07 Other three-wheeled car
08 Taxi
09 Car (four wheeled)
10 Minibus/Motor caravan
11 PSV
12 Goods not over 1 1/2 tons UW (1.52 tonnes)
13 Goods over 1 1/2 tons UW (1.52 tonnes)
14 Other motor vehicle
15 Other non motor vehicle

2.6 Towing and Articulation

`17`

0 No tow/articulation
1 Articulated vehicle
2 Double/multiple trailer
3 Caravan
4 Single trailer
5 Other tow

2.7 Manoeuvres

`18` `19`

01 Reversing
02 Parked
03 Waiting to go ahead but held up
04 Stopping
05 Starting
06 U turn
07 Turning left
08 Waiting to turn left
09 Turning right
10 Waiting to turn right
11 Changing lane to left
12 Changing lane to right
13 Overtaking moving vehicle on its offside
14 Overtaking stationary vehicle on its offside
15 Overtaking on nearside
16 Going ahead left hand bend
17 Going ahead right hand bend
18 Going ahead other

2.8 Vehicle Movement Compass Point

`20` `21`
From To

1 N   2 NE   3 E
4 SE 5 S   6 SW
7 W   8 NW

or `0` `0` Parked - not at kerb

`0` Parked - at kerb

2.9 Vehicle Location at time of Accident

`22` `23`

01 Leaving the main road
02 Entering the main road
03 On main road
04 On minor road
05 On service road
06 On lay-by or hard shoulder
07 Entering lay-by or hard shoulder
08 Leaving lay-by or hard shoulder
09 On a cycleway
10 Not on carriageway

2.10 Junction Location of Vehicle at First Impact

`24`

0 Not at junction (or within 20 metres/22 yards)
1 Vehicle approaching junction/vehicle parked at junction approach
2 Vehicle in middle of junction
3 Vehicle cleared junction/vehicle parked at junction exit
4 Did not impact

2.11 Skidding and Overturning

`25`

0 No skidding, jackknifing or overturning
1 Skidded
2 Skidded and overturned
3 Jackknifed
4 Jackknifed and overturned
5 Overturned

2.12 Hit Object In Carriageway

`26` `27`

00 None
01 Previous accident
02 Road works
03 Parked vehicle - lit
04 Parked vehicle - unlit
05 Bridge (roof)
06 Bridge (side)
07 Bollard/refuge
08 Open door of vehicle
09 Central island or roundabout
10 Kerb
11 Other object

2.13 Vehicle Leaving Carriageway

`28`

0 Did not leave carriageway
1 Left carriageway nearside
2 Left carriageway nearside and rebounded
3 Left carriageway straight ahead at junction
4 Left carriageway offside onto central reservation
5 Left carriageway offside onto central reservation and rebounded
6 Left carriageway offside crossed central reservation
7 Left carriageway offside
8 Left carriageway offside and rebounded

2.14 Hit Object Off Carriageway

`29` `30`

00 None
01 Road sign/Traffic signal
02 Lamp post
03 Telegraph pole/Electricity pole
04 Tree
05 Bus stop/Bus shelter
06 Central crash barrier
07 Nearside or offside crash barrier
08 Submerged in water (completely)
09 Entered ditch
10 Other permanent object

2.15 Vehicle Prefix/Suffix Letter

`31`

Prefix/Suffix letter or one of the following codes -
0 More than twenty years old (at end of year)
1 Unknown/cherished number/not applicable
2 Foreign/diplomatic
3 Military
4 Trade plates

2.16 First Point of Impact

`32`

0 Did not impact
1 Front   2 Back
3 Offside   4 Nearside

2.17 Other Vehicle Hit (VEH Ref No)

`33` `34` `35`

2.18 Part(s) Damaged

`36` `37` `38`

0 None   1 Front
2 Back   3 Offside
4 Nearside   5 Roof
6 Underside   7 all four sides

2.19 No of Axles

`39`

No longer required by the Department of Transport

2.20 Maximum Permissible Gross Weight
Metric tonnes (Goods vehicle only)

`40` `41`

2.21 Sex of Driver

`42`

1 Male   2 Female
3 Not traced

2.22 Age of Driver
(Years estimated if necessary)

`43` `44`

2.23 Breath Test

`45`

0 Not applicable   1 Positive
2 Negative   3 Not requested
4 Failed to provide
5 Driver not contacted at time

2.24 Hit and Run

`46`

0 Other   1 'Hit and run'
2 Non-stop vehicle not hit

2.25 DTp Special Projects

`47` `48` `49` `50`

46

Casualty Record

3.1 Record Type
`[3]` 1 2

1 New casualty record
5 Amended casualty record

3.2 Police Force
`[ ]` 3 4

3.3 Accident Ref No
`[ ]` 5 6 7 8 9 10 11

3.4 Vehicle Ref No
`[ ]` 12 13 14

3.5 Casualty Ref No
`[ ]` 15 16 17

3.6 Casualty Class
`[ ]` 18

1 Driver or Rider
2 Vehicle or pillion passenger
3 Pedestrian

3.7 Sex of Casualty
`[ ]` 19

1 Male
2 Female

3.8 Age of Casualty
`[ ]` 20 21

(Years estimated if necessary)

3.9 Severity of Casualty
`[ ]` 22

1 Fatal
2 Serious
3 Slight

3.10 Pedestrian Location
`[ ]` 23 24

00 Not pedestrian
01 In carriageway crossing on pedestrian crossing
02 In carriageway crossing within zig-zag lines approach to the crossing
03 In carriageway crossing within zig-zag lines exit the crossing
04 In carriageway crossing elsewhere within 50 metres of pedestrian crossing
05 In carriageway crossing elsewhere
06 On footway or verge
07 On refuge or central island or reservation
08 In centre of carriageway not on refuge or central island
09 In carriageway not crossing
10 Unknown

3.11 Pedestrian Movement
`[ ]` 25

0 Not pedestrian
1 Crossing from drivers nearside
2 Crossing from drivers nearside - masked by parked or stationary vehicle
3 Crossing from drivers offside
4 Crossing from drivers offside - masked by parked or stationary vehicle
5 In carriageway stationary - not crossing (standing or playing)
6 In carriageway stationary - not crossing (standing or playing) - masked by parked or stationary vehicle
7 Walking along in carriageway facing traffic
8 Walking along in carriageway back to traffic
9 Unknown

3.12 Pedestrian Direction
`[ ]` 26

Compass point bound

1 N
2 NE
3 E
4 SE
5 S
6 SW
7 W
8 NW
or 0 - Pedestrian - standing still

3.13 School Pupil Casualty
`[ ]` 27

0 Not a school pupil
1 Pupil on journey to/from school
2 Pupil NOT on journey to/from school

3.14 Seat Belt Usage
`[ ]` 28

0 Not car or van
1 Safety belt in use
2 Safety belt fitted - not in use
3 Safety belt not fitted
4 Child safety belt/harness fitted - in use
5 Child safety belt/harness fitted - not in use
6 Child safety belt/harness not fitted
7 Unknown

3.15 Car Passenger
`[ ]` 29

0 Not a car passenger
1 Front seat car passenger
2 Rear seat car passenger

3.16 PSV Passenger
`[ ]` 30

0 Not a PSV passenger
1 Boarding
2 Alighting
3 Standing passenger
4 Seated passenger

3.17 DTp Special Projects
`[ ]` 31 32 33 34